DNA Array Image Analysis
Nuts & Bolts

Edited by

Gerda Kamberova, Ph.D. *and* Shishir Shah, Ph.D.

DNA Press™

Publisher: Xela Schenk
Cover Design and Production Layout: Alex Nartea

ISBN 0-9664027-5-8

Direct all inquiries to DNA Press LLC. For information and mailing address see http://www.dnapress.net

No claim to original U.S. Government works
International Standard Book Number ISBN 0-9664027-5-8
Printed in the United States of America   2 3 4 5 6 7 8 9 0
First printing 2002
Printed on acid-free paper

Contents

Summary of chapters

Chapter 1: Microarrays and Image Analysis: Introduction

The chapter provides brief introduction to microarray technology and the challenges of image analysis in this field. It outlines the objectives of the book. Chapter 1 is intended as a reading material for students and researchers with different scientific backgrounds who are just entering the exciting field of microarray research and applications.

Chapter 2: Introduction to Image Analysis

The chapter introduces basic image analysis terminology and techniques. The digital image, its various representations, and properties are presented. The process of image formation, noise, and noise sources are reviewed. The author discusses important image processing operations. Estimation of image parameters in the presence of noise is addressed. The chapter contains an appendix including mathematical definitions from Fourier analysis and probability theory.

Chapter 3: Advantages of Laser Confocal Microarray Scanning

This chapter provides a general understanding of different approaches used to design commercial microarray scanners. Particular attention is given to laser confocal microarray scanners. Important issues in the authors' discussion are resolution, sensitivity, the use of multiple dyes, and other requirements in the design of commercial microarray scanners.

Chapter 4: Considerations for a Quality Microarray Scanner

This chapter continues the discussion on microarray scanners. Although intended as a general introduction, several features of Agilent's SureScan™ Technology are introduced. The authors discuss issues of instrument noise, sensitivity and resolution.

Chapter 5: Key Considerations for Accurate Microarray Scanning and Image Analysis

This chapter reviews how to obtain the most reliable performance from the microarray scanner. The authors from Axon, Inc. discuss several image analysis methods used in microarray experiments, including numerical pre-processing methods that can be considered prior to cluster analysis of large sets of microarray data.

Chapter 6: Microarray Image Processing and Quality Control

Chapter 6 describes the issues of spot finding, microarray image segmentation, and quality control issues in microarray image analysis. The authors discuss automated batch analysis of microarray images.

Chapter 7: Microarray Data Normalization

This chapter discusses the issue of data normalization for spotted microarrays. The authors dwell on background correction, and data normalization, including a summary of each of the methods which have been widely used. A sample procedure for data normalization is then given along with a brief discussion of types of noise which normalization cannot handle.

Chapter 8: Quantitative Comparison of Image Analysis Software

In this chapter, the authors from Purdue University describe a systematic evaluation of three microarray data acquisition software packages. In order to provide a benchmark to which investigators may compare the reliability of data acquisition in their own experiments, they have evaluated these software packages using a variety of different types of arrays (macro and microarrays; glass and nylon; cDNA and bacterial). The reliability, accuracy, and throughput of data generated from each type of microarray and each software package are discussed.

Chapter 9: DNA Array Information Workflow and Data Management

This chapter outlines the flow of data in a microarray experiment. It discusses some aspects of microarray database management and data mining.

Chapter 10: BAC Microarrays

This chapter discusses an emerging application for microarray technology, which utilizes bacterial artificial chromosomes (BACs). The authors focus on the experimental design, image analysis and data normalization.

Editors

Gerda Kamberova, Ph.D. is an Assistant Professor in Computer Science at Hofstra University, New York. She teaches computer vision, computer graphics, and artificial intelligence. Her Ph.D in Computer Science is from the University of Pennsylvania, Philadelphia. Dr. Kamberova has published research papers in computer vision, robotics, and applied statistics. Her current research interests are in shape representation and recovery and 3D data compression.

Contact:
Gerda L. Kamberova, Ph.D., 103 Hofstra University,
Department of Computer Science, Hempstead, NY 11549 U.S.A.
E-mail: Gerda.L.Kamberova@hofstra.edu

Shishir Shah, Ph.D. is an Associate Professor at Wayne State University (Detroit, MI). Dr. Shah is an author of numerous publications on image analysis and data mining. His current interests are developing new applications for BAC arrays, enhanced microarray image processing and data analysis.

Contact:
Shishir Shah, Ph.D., 2302 Oak Links Avenue,
Houston, TX 77059 U.S.A.
E-mail: sshah@houston.rr.com

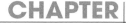
MICROARRAYS AND IMAGE ANALYSIS: INTRODUCTION

Gerda Kamberova, Ph.D. *and* Shishir Shah, Ph.D.

Contact:
Gerda Kamberova, Ph.D.

103 Hofstra University, Department of Computer Science, Hempstead, NY 11549 U.S.A.
E-mail: Gerda.L.Kamberova@hofstra.edu

0-9664027-5-8/02/$0.00+$.50   *From:* **Microarray Image Analysis-Nuts & Bolts** (pp.7-16)
©2002 by DNA Press, LLC   Edited by: S. Shah and G. Kamberova

With the advent of genomics and advanced combinatorial chemistry, large number of compounds and drug targets are now available. Various methods exist for detecting and quantifying gene expression levels, including northern blots[1], differential display[2], sequencing of cDNA libraries[3], S1 nuclease protection[4], and serial analysis of gene expressions[5]. Over the last several years there has been an explosion of microarray technology in the biosciences, medical sciences, biotechnology, and pharmaceutical industry. The technology has centered on providing a platform for determining, in a single experiment, the gene expression profiles of hundreds to tens of thousands of genes (or transcript levels of RNA species) in tissue, tumors, cells, or biological fluids. The rapid and global adoption of this technology has been predicated on its simplicity and success in providing large amounts of highly relevant data. Gene expression microarrays is the key technology to alleviate the bottleneck in drug discovery and disease diagnostics. Microarrays can easily determine the expression of thousands of genes. As the demand to conduct analysis on a genome-wide basis increases, the challenges for improved data extraction and analysis are growing. There are now hundreds of published papers in the literature on microarrays and the application of microarray technology in biological research.

1.1 Microarrays

In their most generic form, microarrays are ordered sets of DNA molecules attached to a solid surface. Hundreds to tens of thousands molecules are organized in a two dimensional array (matrix). The DNA molecules are typically either oligonucleotide (ranging form 35 base pairs to several hundred) or cDNAs. The matrix to which the DNA molecule is attached is usually glass, silicon, or nylon. Before the DNA is spotted, the matrix is typically coated with a material such as poly-lysine, silane, or other chemicals to make the matrix reactive. In most cases, the DNA is attached to it using UV radiation or covalent coupling to permanently link the DNA to the surface. In this form a cDNA or oligonucleotide, corresponding to a specific sequence of a gene, can be spotted onto the solid surface. That can be repeated for hundreds to tens of thousands of genes. With this set of DNA segments attached to the surface, RNA from a specimen (e.g. tissue, cell line, tumor) can be labeled directly or indirectly (usually with a fluorescent nucleotide) and hybridized to the array of genes. The amount of fluorescence at each DNA spot corresponds to the transcript level of that particular gene. Therefore, the expression of thousands of genes can be analyzed in a single specimen by analyzing the image of a microarray.

From an information processing perspective, microarray technology aids the researcher in transforming and supplementing data available on genes and cells into useful information about gene expression, and ultimately, cellular biology. Microarrays allow one to study expression levels in parallel. The hybridization between nucleic acids when one of them is fixed within a matrix forms the basis of many experimental analysis in molecular biology. This method provides excellent detection due to mutual selectivity between complementary strands of nucleic acids. Most experiments of this method used to employ a single labeled oligonucleotide or polynucleotide species in a liquid phase attached to a solid transport. Transcript abundance is assayed by immobilizing mRNA or total RNA on membranes and then incubating with a radioactively labeled gene-specific target. If multiple mRNA samples are immobilized on the same matrix, one obtains information about the quantity of a particular message present in each RNA pool. cDNA arrays experiments use many gene-specific polynucleotides derived from the ends of RNA transcripts. These are arrayed on a single matrix and simultaneously probed with a fluorescently tagged cDNA representation of total RNA pools from test and reference cells. One can determine the relative amount of transcript present in the pool by the type of fluorescent signal generated. The relative message abundance is based on a comparison of the test cell state to a reference cell state. The scheme is similar to using radiolabeled probes, but it is not possible to carry out simultaneous hybridization of test and reference samples. Serial or parallel hybridization can be used to overcome this limitation. Initial work by Kozal, Chee, Lockhart, and others [6,7,8,9,10] demonstrated the power of this technology for genomic research. Affymetrix pioneered the approach of synthesizing oligonucleotides onto a solid substrate using photolithographic techniques. Due to the cost and complexity of this technology, many researchers explored alternative methods, most notably the groups of Pat Brown and Ron Davis at Stanford University[6]. The alternative technology involves the printing of DNA onto a solid substrate and then probing it with labeled DNA sequences. The microarray technology provides an unprecedented means for carrying out high-throughput gene expression analysis experiments.

1.2 Microarray Image Processing

Images record and represent visual information. In engineering and science, image processing is used to examine properties of objects or processes encoded in images. Tendencies of the objects or processes under study are recoded in the images, and the goal of image analysis it to extract and quantify these tendencies. Examples of image analysis tasks performed by computer systems are: optical character recognition, such as reading ZIP codes or hand written checks; detecting, outlining, and measuring objects, like boundaries of blood vessels, structural deformations of the heart, degeneration of the retina, in medical applications; and extracting spots and detecting their boundaries, and then estimating parameters which quantify gene expression levels in microarray applications.

The main classes of problems addressed in digital image processing are: image representation and modeling, image enhancement, image restoration, image analysis, and image data compression. Image enhancement improves the quality of images (for example, by increasing the contrast). It is usually performed as a preprocessing step in many image processing and computer vision tasks. Image restoration, or cleaning, removes or suppresses discrepancies or undesirable features that appear in the image. Such features are called noise. Related problems are noise removal or noise suppression. Image segmentation methods partition the image into different, non-overlapping regions, based on certain attributes. Examples of attributes are brightness, color, or surface markings. Image segmentation is one of the most fundamental image analysis tasks. Segmentation problems are also among the most difficult in general cases. Feature extraction identifies and labels features of interest in the image. In various applications features may be regions, blobs, contour boundaries of objects, corners, specific geometric shapes, faces of people, cars, planes, or other objects of interest. Usually, segmentation precedes feature extraction.

During the image analysis process, image enhancement, segmentation, background and feature extraction, and statistical methods and procedures are used to infer and quantify parameters characterizing the objects or processes being studied. Information about the parameters is usually indirectly recorded in the image. The difficulties in quantifying parameter values are amplified by the presence of noise in the images. Thus, in addition to quantifying the parameters, in many applications in medicine, engineering, or science, it is necessary not only to measure the parameters, but also to specifying the accuracy and the precision of the measurements, i.e. to assess the quality of the estimates.

The fundamental goal of microarray image processing is to measure the intensities of the arrayed spots, and based on these intensities to quantify the spots expression levels. In a more sophisticated and complete approach, the array image processing will also assess the reliability of the quantified spot data and generate warnings to the possible problems during the array production and/or hybridization phases.

1.3 Microarray Image Analysis: Properties, Problems, and Main Tasks

Microarray images consist of arrays of spots, also referred to as grids, arranged in a prespecified matrix. Typically, all the grids have the same numbers of rows and columns of spots. These grids, called "sub-grids", are arranged in relatively equal spacing with each other, forming a "meta-array". This meta-array structure is formed by using a robotic arraying system which uses multiple "pins" to create the array. Each pin deposits DNA material in a single sub-grid.

Ideally, the microarray images should have the following properties:

- All the sub-grids are the same size.
- The spacing between the sub-grids is regular.
- The distance between adjacent rows and columns in a sub-grid is the same.
- The location of the spots is centered on the intersections of the lines of the rows and columns.
- The spot shape is a perfect circle, and the spot size is constant.
- For a given type of slides, the grid position is fixed over multiple images.
- No dust or other contamination is present on the slide.
- There are minimal undesirable artifacts (noise) in the images.
- The background intensity is uniform across the image.

If all these idealized conditions were satisfied, the image processing task could be accomplished by a simple computer program. An array of circles with the defined dimensions and spacing can be superimposed on the image. The areas falling inside these circles would be considered signal (spots) and the outside area would be background. However, most, if not all, of these idealized conditions are often violated. These violations may be conceptualized as four issues: spot position variation, spot shape and size irregularity, noise and contamination, and global problems that are affecting multiple spots.

The main tasks in microarray image analysis are:

- Noise suppression.
- Spot localization and detection, including the extraction of the background intensity, the spot position, and the spot boundary and size.
- Data quantification and quality assessment.

Here we summarize the steps. After introducing necessary definitions and techniques from image analysis in Chapter 2, all tasks are discussed in detail in later chapters of the book.

1.3.1 Spot Localization and Image Segmentation

The goal of the spot finding operation is to locate the spots (signal) in images and estimate the size of each spot. Based on the degree of human intervention, there are three levels of sophistication in the algorithms for spot finding, these are discussed in Chapter 6. The ultimate goal of array image processing is to build an automatic system, which utilizes computer vision algorithms, to find the spots without the need for any human intervention. This method would greatly reduce the human effort, minimize the potential for human error, and offer a great deal of consistency in the quality of data. Such a processing system would require the user to specify the expected configuration of the array (e.g., number of rows and columns of spots), and would automatically search the image for the grid position. Having found the approximate grid position, which specify the center of each spot, the spot neighborhood can be examined.

A small patch around that location (target region) can be used to quantify the spot expression level. The next step is to determine which pixels in the target region are due to the actual spot signal and which are background. At this stage, the size and shape irregularities of the spots and any contamination problem in the images are the major concern to the algorithm design. Knowledge about the image characteristics should be incorporated to account for variabilities in microarray images. The spot location, size, and shape should be adjusted to accommodate for noise and contamination. A number of methods have been developed. The advantages and disadvantages of these methods are described by *Petrov et al.* in Chapter 6 of this book.

1.3.2 Data Quantification

Once the spots are located, and signal and background segmented, various parameters are estimated using the intensity of the segmented regions. These parameters are *total, mean, median, mode,* and *volume* of the intensity in the regions, and *intensity ratio* and *correlation ratio* across two channels. The underlying principle for judging which parameter to use is based on how well each of these measurements correlates to the amount of the DNA probe present at the spots.

The key information that needs to be recorded from microarrays is the expression strength of each target spot. In gene expression studies, one is typically interested in the difference in expression levels between the test and reference mRNA populations. This translates in differences in the intensities of the reference and target images. Under idealized conditions, the total florescent intensity from a spot is proportional to the expression strength. These idealized conditions imply that the preparation of the probe cDNA solution and the hybridization are done appropriately; the exact amount of cDNA is deposited on each spot during the chip fabrication; there is no contamination over the spots; and that the spot pixels are correctly identified by image analysis. Even if the preparation and hybridization are done properly, the rest of the conditions are often violated. The DNA concentrations in the spotting procedure may vary temporally and spatially. Higher concentrations may result in larger spot sizes. When spots are contaminated, the intensity over the contaminated region cannot be measured accurately. The image processing may not correctly identify all the signal pixels, thus, quantification methods should be designed to address these problems.

1.3.3 Quality Measurements

Important steps in processing microarray images are the assessment of the reliability of the data obtained and the report of possible problems with the images. Without these the conclusions drawn from the data may be incorrect leading to a false hypothesis, or an omission of important findings. The reliability of the data is affected by multiple factors, ranging from problems in the array fabrication and the experimental setup to problems in the image processing. The quality control may be performed by a human operator, or by image processing software. In a high-throughput gene expression analysis system the quality assessment needs to be done automatically, by software.

1.4 Data Analysis and Visualization Techniques

The image processing and analysis step produces a large number of quantified gene expression levels. The data typically represents thousands or tens of thousands of gene expression levels across multiple experiments. To make sense of so much data, it is unavoidable to use various visualization and statistical analysis techniques. One of the typical microarray data analysis goals is to find statistically significantly up or down regulated genes, in other words outliers or 'interestingly' behaving genes in the data[11]. Another possible goal would be to find functional groupings of genes by discovering similarity or dissimilarity among gene expression profiles, or predicting the biochemical and physiological pathways of previously uncharacterized genes[12]. The main approaches to data analysis and visualization are scatter plots, principal components analysis, cluster analysis, and data normalization and transformation.

1.5 New Developments and Challenges of the Microarray Technology

The maturation process of microarray technology has brought new applications. One of them is the array CGH (Comparative Genomic Hybridization) methodology. The introduction of CGH to metaphase chromosomes revolutionized the clinical cytogenetics diagnostic arena by permitting the genome wide analysis of cancer specimens with chromosomal aberrations that were either too many or too complex to be fully characterized by routine cytogenetics[13]. Moreover, since CGH required only genomic DNA from the specimen sample, it permitted the analysis of specimens from which chromosomal preparations were either impractical or impossible. However, the use of metaphase chromosomes as the platform against which the CGH was performed meant that the inherent resolution levels associated with metaphase chromosomes persisted. In practice, this meant that CGH to metaphase chromosomes remained largely incapable of accomplishing genome-wide screens for chromosomal aberrations that were less than about 5 Mb, a limitation which made this approach unsuitable for detecting many of the non-cancer-related genetic aberrations encountered in the routine day-to-day portfolio of a clinical cytogenetics laboratory. Recently, with the advent of bacterial artificial chromosome (BAC) array technology and the ability to screen the entire genome, has re-drawn the attention to the applicability of CGH, albeit array CGH, in the routine cytogenetics laboratory. So-called array or matrix CGH utilizes mapped DNA sequences in a microarray format as an alternative platform for the CGH analysis. Hence, the resolution level of this approach is dependent on a combination of the number, size and map positions of the DNA elements within the array. In recent years, several reports have described adaptation of microarray technology to the study of genomic alterations[14]. Unfortunately, these technologies have been difficult to adapt to clinical and research laboratories. Recently, the advent of BAC arrays (Spectral Genomics, Inc., Houston, TX) has yielded high-resolution genomic scans (currently at 1 Mb) in a rapid and highly reproducible fashion. Testing has begun on the suitability of the BAC array approach with commercially available human genome arrays for incorporation into the day-to-day repertoire of cytogenetic diagnostic procedures. A number of clinical specimens as well as cell lines with a broad spectrum of known constitutional and acquired genetic aberrations were chosen for the study, the results of which, conclusively demonstrate the evolving position of microarray genome profiling as an indispensable addition to the repertoire of cytogenetic diagnostic procedures. The last chapter of this book is devoted to BAC array technology and its applications to biology and medicine.

The progress in microarray technology has solved some of the initial challenges of this high throughput screening methodology. One such challenge is to develop the hardware for conducting hybridization experiments. The other is to manage the massive amount of information associated with this technology, so that the results can yield understandings to the genomic functions in biological systems. With the steady progress of the developments of the hardware technology, currently available equipment can reliably produce an image on the order of 40,000 and more spots on a single microscope slide. In other words, the fundamental challenge from hardware has been mostly resolved.

On the other hand, the informatics challenge has just emerged. There are three major issues involved. The first is to keep track of the information generated at the stages of chip production and hybridization experiment. The second is to process microarray images to obtain the quantified gene expression values from the arrays. The third is to mine the information from the gene expression data. As the final hypothesis verification is based on the outcome of data analysis, it is imperative that the computations performed in the image analysis steps are reliable and that they provide repetitive unbiased estimates.

References

1. *Alwine JC, Kemp DJ, Stark GR*: Method for detection of specific RNAs in agarose gels by transfer to diazobenzyloxymethyl-paper and hybridization with DNA probes. *PNAS U.S.A.*, 1977; 74:5350-5354.

2. *Liang P, Pardee AB*: Differential display of eukaryotic messenger RNA by means of polymerase chain reaction. *Science 1992*; 257:967-971.

2. *Okubo K*: Large-scale cDNA sequencing for analysis of quantitative and qualitative aspects of gene expression. *Nature Genetics* 1992; 2:173-179.

3. *Berk AJ, Sharp PA*: Sizing and mapping of early adenovirus mRNAs by gel electrophoresis of S1 endonuclease-digested hybrids. *Cell 1977*; 12:721-732.

4. *Velculescu VE, Zhang L, Vogelstein B, Kinzler KW*: Serial analysis of gene expression. *Science* 1995; 270:484-487.

5. *Brown PO, Botstein D*: Exploring the new world of the genome with DNA microarrays. *Nature Genetics Supplement* 1999; 21:33-37.

6. *Fodor SPA, Stryer L, Read JL, Pirrung MC*: Array of materials attached to a substrate. *U.S. Patent 5,744,305*, 1998.

7. *Hacia JG*: Resequencing and mutational analysis using oligonucleotide microarrays. *Nature Genetics Supplement* 1999; 21:42-47.

8. *Kozal MJ, Shah N, Shen N, Yang R, Fucini R, Merigan TC, Richman DD, Morris D, Hubbell E, Chee M, Gingeras TR*: Extensive polymorphisms observed in HIV-1 clade B potease gene using high-density oligonucleotide arrays. *Nature Medicine* 1996; 2:253-257.

9. *Woodicka L, Dong H, Mittman M, Ho M-H, Lockhart DJ*: Genome wide expression monitoring in Saccharomyces cerevisiae. *Nature Biotechnology* 1999; 15:1359,-1362

10. *Heyer LJ, Kruglyak S, Yooseph S*: Exploring Expression Data: Identification and Analysis of coexpressed Genes. *Genome Res* 1999; 9:1106-1115.

11. **Hilsenbeck SG, Friedrichs WE, Schiff R, O'Connell P, Hansen RK, Osborne CK, Fuqua SAW**: Statistical Analysis of Array Expression Data as Applied to the Problem of Tamoxifen Resistance. *Journal of the National Cancer Institute* 1999; 91(5):453-459.

12. **Kirchhoff M, Rose H, Lundsteen C**: High Resolution Comparative Genomic Hybridization in Clinical Cytogenetics, *J of Med Genetics* 2001; 38(11):740-744.

13. **Pollack JR, Perou CM, Alizadeh AA, Eisen MB, Pergamenschikov A, Williams CF, Jeffrey SS, Botstein D, Brown PO:** Genome-wide Analysis of DNA Copy-number Changes Using cDNA Microarrays. *Nature Genetics* 1999; 23: 41-46.

14. **Pinkel D, Segraves R, Sudor D, Clark S, Poole I, Kowbel D, Collins C, Kuo WL, Chen C, Zhai Y, Dairkee SH, Ljung BM, Gray JW, Albertson DG**: High Resolution Analysis of DNA Copy Number Variation Using Comparative Genomic Hybridization to Microarrays. *Nature Genetics* 1998; 20:207-211.

CHAPTER
2

INTRODUCTION TO IMAGE ANALYSIS

Gerda Kamberova, Ph.D.

Contact:
Gerda Kamberova, Ph.D.

103 Hofstra University, Department of Computer Science, Hempstead, NY 11549 U.S.A.
E-mail: Gerda.L.Kamberova@hofstra.edu

0-9664027-5-8/02/$0.00+$.50   *From:* **Microarray Image Analysis-Nuts & Bolts** (pp.17-50)
©2002 by DNA Press, LLC   Edited by: S. Shah and G. Kamberova

2.1 Introduction

The objective of this chapter is to introduce the image analysis terminology and techniques that are relevant to microarray applications, and thus to provide a foundation for understanding later chapters of this book.

The main classes of problems addressed in digital image processing are: image representation and modeling, image enhancement, image restoration, image analysis, and image data compression[1]. *Image enhancement* improves the quality of images (for example increases contrast). It is performed usually as a preprocessing step in many image processing and computer vision tasks. *Image restoration*, or cleaning, removes or suppresses discrepancies or undesirable features that appear in the image. Such features are called *noise*. Related problems are *noise removal* or *noise suppression*. *Image segmentation* methods partition the image into different, non-overlapping regions based on certain attributes. Examples of attributes are brightness, color, or surface markings. Image segmentation is one of the most fundamental image analysis tasks. Segmentation problems are also among the most difficult in general cases. *Feature extraction* identifies and labels features of interest in the image. Examples of features are regions, blobs, contour boundaries of objects, corners, specific geometric shapes, faces of people, cars, planes, or other objects of interest in various applications. Usually, segmentation precedes feature extraction. In *image analysis* image enhancement, segmentation, background and feature extraction, and statistical methods and procedures are used to infer and quantify parameters of interest characterizing objects or processes under study.

The images studied and analyzed in this book are images of microarrays. The goal is to obtain quantitative measures of gene expressions present in the printed microarray. The methods employed are segmentation, boundary extraction, and statistical inferences. This chapter is organized as follow: first we discuss what a computer image is; next we introduce image models (as spatial functions, as linear combination of basis functions, as stochastic processes, and as linear systems); then we present color models and basic properties of digital images; after that, we summarize fundamental image operations, and discuss the image quality and noise. As a Supplement we include a section with mathematical definitions related to the Fourier transform and probability theory.

2.2 The Computer Image

2.2.1 Bits and Pixels

Most people think of a computer image as a picture they see on the display, Figure 2-1.

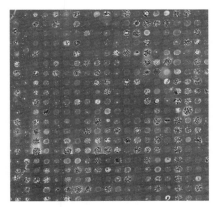

Figure 2-1. Part from a microarray image (courtesy of BioDiscovery, Inc). This particular section shows perfectly circular spots together with problems in the image such as dust particles in some spots and in the background area, as well as streaks over the spots.

Internally, a computer image is a two-dimensional array of numbers. An image of size M x N is an array **f** of M rows and N columns,

$$\mathbf{f} = \{f(x,y): x = 0,1,...,M-1, y = 0,1,...,N-1\}$$

For monochromatic images $f(x,y)$ is an integer number, called a *gray value*. It can take one of a finite set of values of a *gray scale*. Each $f(x,y)$ represents the brightness (intensity) of a small picture element, called pixel, at location (x,y), see Figure 2-2. In Figure 2-2(a) a pixel is represented as one of the small squares. A pixel has a location, (x,y), a value, $f(x,y)$, and also a size, $\Delta x \times \Delta y$, the area of the small rectangle (square). In case of color images, $f(x,y)$ is a vector (triplet of numbers). Each triplet represents one color. Often the word pixel is used to denote not only the picture element, but also its location and its value. Computer images are most often called *digital images*. Next we discuss how a digital image is stored in the computer memory.

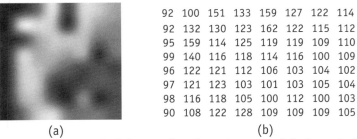

92	100	151	133	159	127	122	114
92	132	130	123	162	122	115	112
95	159	114	125	119	119	109	110
99	140	116	118	114	116	100	109
96	122	121	112	106	103	104	102
97	121	123	103	101	103	105	104
98	116	118	105	100	112	100	103
90	108	122	128	109	109	109	105

(a)   (b)

Figure 2-2. **(a)** An image detail of size 8x8 pixels from the center of the image in Figure 2-1, enlarged 48 times; and **(b)** the internal representation of the detail as an array of numbers. Each number represents the gray level at the corresponding pixel in (a). Higher values in (b) are displayed with lighter shades of gray in (a). The size of the image in Figure 2-1 is 391x391 pixels.

19

In everyday life people use numbers represented in the Decimal number system. The radix is 10, any number is a linear combination of powers of 10, and it is written as a sequence of the decimal digits, 0 to 9. For example,

$$129 = 1 \times 10^2 + 2 \times 10^1 + 9 \times 10^0.$$

Unlike people, computers use the Binary number system. A number that is stored in the computer memory is represented in binary, i.e., as a sequence of zeros and ones.

The computer memory consists of cells called bytes. A byte contains eight *bits* (for short from *bi*nary dig*its*). Any number can be represented in the Binary number system. The radix is 2, the number is represented as linear combination of powers of 2, and it is written as a sequence of the binary digits, 0 and 1. For example,

$$129 = 1 \times 2^7 + 0 \times 2^6 + 0 \times 2^5 + 0 \times 2^4 + 0 \times 2^3 + 0 \times 2^2 + 0 \times 2^1 + 1 \times 2^0.$$

In the Binary number system the number 129 is represented by the sequence 10000001,

$$10000001_{(2)} = 129_{(10)}$$

A bit can hold one binary digit, 0 or 1, so a sequence of binary digits is stored into a sequence of bits, and so is a pixel value.

A *one-bit digital image* is an image for which the computer uses one bit to represent a pixel value. A one-bit image is also called a *binary image*. In a binary image a pixel value could be either 0 (black) or 1 (white). In a *two-bit image*, two bits are used per pixel value. The possible binary sequences of length two are 00, 01, 10, and 11. Thus only four possible gray levels can appear, black (00), white (11) and two shades of gray (01 and 10). And in an *n* -bit image, *n* bits are used to represent a pixel value. Since there are 2^n possible binary sequences of length *n*, a pixel can have one of 2^n possible values.

A typical monochromatic image is 8-bit, so a pixel can have one of 256 possible gray levels. The decimal number 0 (the sequence of eight binary 0's) corresponds to black, and the decimal number 255 (a sequence of eight binary 1's) corresponds to white, and there are 254 gray levels in between. A typical color image is 24-bit. We come back to color images when we discuss color models.

Next we consider important attributes of digital images, namely the radiometric and the spatial resolutions.

2.2.2 Radiometric and Spatial Resolutions of a Digital Image

The *radiometric resolution* of a digital image is given by the number of bits used per pixel value, and it limits the maximal number of gray levels or colors that can be represented in the image. It is measured in bits/pixel. Images of low radiometric resolution may exhibit false contours when displayed. The *spatial resolution* of a digital image is given by the number of pixels per unit area, and it limits the size of the smallest detail that could be distinguished in the image. Images of low spatial resolution may appear blocky when displayed, the individual pixels (squares) are visible. Compare the image in Figure 2-2(a), of low spatial resolution, with the image in Figure 2-1, of high spatial resolution. Later we discuss the spatial and radiometric resolution of video sensors.

2.3 Image Models

Here we overview the mathematical models used in image analysis. We limit the discussion to monochromatic images. The treatment of color images is similar. We have included a Supplement to the chapter with a brief summary of the mathematics needed.

2.3.1 Images as Two-dimensional Intensity Functions

A continuous image can be modeled as a function, $z = f(x,y)$, of two independent variables. The real coordinates x and y specify location in the xy-plane, and the image intensity $f(x,y)$ represents height z above the xy-plane, Figure 2-3. Thus the image is considered a two-dimensional surface consisting of the three-dimensional points with coordinates $(x,y,f(x,y))$. Although this is not the natural way people think of images, it is a representation that is useful computationally. A digital image approximates a continuous one, and the surface points for digital images, $(x,y,f(x,y))$, have only integer coordinates. For an n -bit digital image of size $M \times N$,

$$x = 0,1,...,M-1, \quad y = 0,1,...,N-1, \quad \text{and} \quad 0 \le f(x,y) \le 2^n - 1.$$

A representation of an image as an intensity function, $f(x,y)$, of two coordinates in a spatial planar domain (i.e. the coordinates x and y identify locations) is called *spatial-domain representation*. There are other image representations that have computational advantages for image processing. Next we explore one such representation, the frequency-domain representation using basis functions.

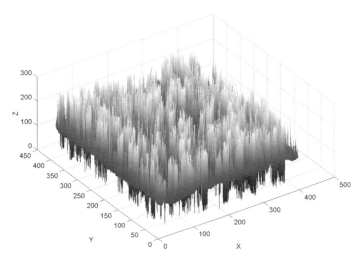

Figure 2-3. The image from Figure 2-1 displayed as a spatial function $z = f(x,y)$.

2.3.2 Image Representation Through Basis Functions

In image processing, images traditionally are represented by series expansions in two-dimensional orthogonal functions called basis functions (or basis images). The term orthogonal basis has a precise mathematical meaning, but for our discussion, it suffices to say that the collection of the basis functions is such that they are all essential, i.e., none of them can be expressed in terms of the rest, and any digital image can be represented uniquely as a weighted sum of the basis functions. The coefficients that weight the basis function in the sum comprise the new image representation, called *frequency-domain representation*. The mappings from spatial domain-representation to frequency-domain representation are called image transforms. There is a highly developed mathematical theory to study various image properties using image transforms, and there are very efficient methods for computing with them. Problems that rely heavily by on image transforms are filter design, feature extraction, and image compression. The classical approach to filter design is based on the *Fourier transform*, which we review in the Supplement 2A. Using a discrete Fourier transform, a digital image is represented as a weighted sum of two-dimensional sinusoidal functions, i.e., the basis functions are sinusoidal functions of two independent variables. The Fourier theory prescribes how to compute the weights corresponding to the basis functions. In the last ten, fifteen years *wavelet transforms* have gained popularity in image analysis. Their use has certain advantages over the Fourier transform for multi-resolution filter design and image compression[3].

2.3.3 Images as Random Fields

Another useful model of digital images is based on probability theory. A digital image is viewed as a realization of a random (stochastic) process,[6]. The randomness arises due to uncertainty in the environment and the physics of the video sensors. When an image is considered as a realization of a stochastic process, it is described as a member of a whole class of possible images. In this model, a *random variable*, Z_{xy}, is associated with each pixel site. The two-dimensional array of these random variables is called a *spatial stochastic process*, also called a *random field*,

$$Z = \{Z_{xy} : x = 0,1,...,M -1, y = 0,1,...,N -1\}.$$

A particular image, z, is and observation (a sample) from the random field, Z,

$$z = \{z_{xy} : x = 0,1,...,M -1, y = 0,1,...,N -1\},$$

where z is the array of pixel values.

A random field is characterized by the *joint probability distribution function*, $F_Z(z)$, or the *joint probability density function*, $f_Z(z)$ of all random variables that comprise it. (Definitions from probability theory are summarized at the end of the Supplement 2A.) The *mean* of the random field is the two-dimensional array (a matrix) with elements the expected values of the random variables at the individual pixel sites,

$$E[Z] = \{E[Z_{xy}] : x = 0,1,...,M -1, y = 0,1,...,N -1\}.$$

The *covariance* of the random field is a matrix that has an element for each pair of pixel sites, each element equals the covariance between the random variables at the pixel sites of the pair.

To prescribe a stochastic model for a class of n-bit digital images, it is not practical to list explicitly the value of the probability density for each possible image, since the number of possible images is huge, $2^n MN$. For an 8-bit image of size 1024 by 1024 this is of the order of a billion images. Thus, simplifications are made. Often it is assumed that the random field is a *second order process*, i.e., it is completely specified in terms of its first and second moments[1]. The means of the individual random variables and the covariances between any two of them are given by the mean and covariance functions, $\mu(x,y)$, $r(x,y,p,q)$, i.e., for values of $x,p = 0,1,...,M -1$, $y,q = 0,1,...,N -1$, the corresponding elements of the mean and covariance matrices of the process are

$$E[Z_{xy}] = \mu(x,y), \quad Cov[Z_{xy},Z_{pq}] = r(x,y,p,q).$$

A *stationary random field* is a second-order spatial process for which the mean and covariance functions do not depend on the actual pixel locations, i.e., the stationary property specifies some global spatial properties of the image. For a stationary process, the mean of the process has the same elements at all sites, and the covariance between two random variables at two pixel sites depends only on the relative (not actual) position of the pixels. Thus for a stationary random field, the mean is constant, and the covariance is completely characterized by a covariance matrix with elements $Cov[Z_{xy}, Z_{00}]$, where x and y vary over the rows and columns of the image. Both, the mean and the covariance, matrices have the same size, and it is equal to the size of the image. A *white noise random field* is a second order process with uncorrelated elements, i.e., any two variables from the random field are uncorrelated. A *Gaussian random field* is a second order process for which the collection of any subset of random variables from the field has a joint Gaussian (normal) distribution.

A *markov random field* (MRF) is a random field in which the probability that a pixel at site (x,y) has some value, given the rest of the image, actually depends only on the values of close by pixels. MRF are characterized by local spatial dependencies in the image. Often stationary MRF are used to specify images since they are easy to prescribe in term of *local characteristics* (probabilities over a neighborhood, not the whole image grid)[14]. In fact any random field is a markov random field, but of interests are only those models that have small enough neighborhoods to be computationally tractable, and yet are expressive enough to model rich classes of images.

The random field representations of images are used in image restoration, feature extraction, image segmentation, noise reduction, and parameter estimation[1]. For example, one approach to image restoration is to infer the characteristic of a true, unobservable image x, from the observed image z which is a sample from a random field Z. *Wiener filtering* is an image restoration procedure that uses stationary Gaussian white noise model for inferring x. Various statistical methods are used for making inferences (estimates). Some of these methods are least squares estimation, minimum mean square methods, maximum likelihood, Bayesian estimation, including maximum a posteriori (MAP) estimation, and Gibbs sampler techniques, autoregression (AR). Of increasing interest are the robust statistical procedures, which give stable estimates even when the data deviate from the models adopted.

2.3.4 Images as Linear Systems

An imaging system, or an image analysis procedure, can be modeled as a *two-dimensional linear system* H. Such a system takes a sequence of two-dimensional input signals, and produces an output sequence of two-dimensional signals. A *two-dimensional signal* is a function of two independent variables, for example an image. If f denotes the input signal, and g, the output one, the system is written as

$$g = H[f].$$

The system is *linear shift-invariant*, if it preserves linear combinations and translations, i.e., for every choice of the coordinates (x,y), and the numbers a_1, a_2, a, and b, the following properties of linearity and shifting hold,

$$H[a_1 f_1(x,y)+a_2 f_2(x,y)] = a_1 H[f_1(x,y)]+a_2 H[f_2(x,y)],$$

$$H[f(x-a,y-b)] = g(x-a,y-b).$$

The signals could be represented using the spatial- or the frequency-domain approach. In the spatial-domain representation a linear shift-invariant system is completely specified by its *impulse response*, h, and in the frequency-domain by its *transfer function H*. This means that if the impulse response, or equivalently, the transfer function of the system is specified, the output from the system for any input can be calculated. In the spatial-domain the system output g is the *convolution* of the input f with impulse response h,

$$g(x,y) = f(x,y)*h(x,y),$$

and in the frequency-domain, the output G it is the product of the input F with the transfer function H,

$$G(u,v) = F(u,v)H(u,v).$$

The impulse response of the system and the transfer function are a *Fourier transform pair*, they are two different representations of the same linear shift-invariant system, one in the spatial- and the other in the frequency-domain. The Fourier transform, the convolution operator, and related properties are given in the Supplement 2A. A discrete version and applications of the convolution are presented farther in the chapter. For optical imaging systems, the impulse response prescribes how an image of a point light source in the input is smeared in the output image. For that reason the impulse response in such systems is called point-spread function. Linear systems are divided into two categories based in their impulse responses, finite impulse response (FIR) and infinite impulse response (IIR) systems[1].

2.3.5 Filtering

Linear shift-invariant systems are extensively used in *filter design* problems. Filtering is a fundamental image processing operation. The action of the system on the input is called *filtering*. The impulse response and the transfer function of the system are called spatial and frequency filters, respectively. The objective of the filter design is, given the type of desired outputs, to construct the impulse response or transfer function specifying the linear shift-invariant system that generates such outputs, i.e., given what features of the input should be present in the output, to come up with the proper $h(x,y)$ or $H(x,y)$. Spatial filters are designed in the spatial domain, and frequency filters in the frequency domain. For computational reasons the frequency-domain filtering is predominant.

Equipped with image representation models, we are ready to discuss the video sensor and the image formation process.

2.4 The Image Formation: Sampling, Quantization, Noise Sources

2.4.1 Image Formation

Depending on the light source imaging techniques are classified into *passive* and *active*. In passive techniques, sources of light are already present in the environment, and are not part of the imaging system. The human vision system and TV cameras are examples of passive vision systems.

In active imaging techniques, the energy source is part of the system. Such system can control the source of the radiation. The active imaging systems are predominant in medical and biological fields. Examples of such system include laser range finders, MRI scanners, and microarry scanners.

Typically, a digital image is obtained using a CCD camera system, which consists of: optics (lens), a CCD array with photosensitive elements (called *sels*[7]), and an analog-to-digital converter (ADC). The ADC is on the chip for digital cameras, and it is in an external frame-grabber (digitizer) for analog CCD cameras.

The process of digital image formation can be described roughly as follows. Light collected by the lens falls onto the sel array. The photons excite electrons, and electrical charges are collected into "potential wells" at the sel sites, next the charges are transferred (in scan line order) and measured to produce the pixel values[8]. Thus the process is from photons to electric charges (analog), and to pixels (digital).

Images that are formed on a high quality photographic film may be considered continuous. Points in the image are infinitely close together, their locations are denoted by real numbers, and also the intensity value at a point is a nonnegative real number. Digital images are obtained by scanning continuous images or through direct observation of the continuous world with video sensors. The processes that are used to form digital images from continuous signals are *sampling* and *quantization*. The sampling defines the *spatial resolution*, and the quantization, the *radiometric resolution* of the video sensor, or the digital images obtained with the sensor.

2.4.2 Sampling

The output from an analog CCD camera is a one-dimensional analog signal, and an external ADC is used to sample it and assemble it into two-dimensional digital image. In a digital CCD camera this process is done on the chip. In either case, a video sensor samples a continuous signal into a discrete format. *Sampling* is the process of measuring the continuous signal $f(x,y)$ at discrete intervals in the xy-plane, and *quantization*, at discrete intervals in intensity, the z axis, (refer to Figure 2-3). The sampling rate defines the number of pixels per unit area, and thus the spatial resolution of the image. The spatial resolution of an imaging sensor could be defined also as the spatial intervals at which samples (measurements) of the continuous function are taken. The *sampling rate* limits the spatial resolution. With high sampling rate, the samples are taken at small intervals, which leads to a high-resolution digital image (large number of pixels of small size each). With low sampling rate, the samples are taken at large intervals, which leads to a low-resolution image (small number of pixels of large individual sizes). The sampling rate of a video sensor should be high enough to preserve desirable level of detail in the image.

2.4.3 Sampling Rate and the Nyquist Limit

The rate of intensity change in an image is measured by the spatial frequency. Graduate changes in brightness are characterized by low spatial frequencies, and sharp changes, by high spatial frequencies. In order for a digital image to represent faithfully the original signal from which it was obtained, the sampling rate of the video sensor has to be at least twice the highest spatial frequency present in the original signal. That condition is known as the *Nyquist theorem*. The frequency that is half the sampling rate of a video sensor is called the *Nyquist limit*. If the original signal contains spatial frequencies above the Nyquist limit, these frequencies will not be recorded properly: any changes in intensity higher than 0.5 cycles per pixel will be lost or severely distorted in the digital image. Such discrepancies are called *aliasing*. Since usually it is not possible to know in advance the highest spatial frequencies that may appear in input signals, sampling is preceded by antialiasing (removing from the original signal spatial frequencies that are higher than the Nyquist limit). With antialiasing, small size detail will be lost, but severe distortions, not present in the original signal, will not appear in the digital image.

2.4.4 Quantization

In addition to discretizing spatially the continuous signal, video sensors discretize the continuous range of signal values (i.e., the light intensity). This process is known as quantization. The range of possible values of the continuous intensity function is replaced by a finite number of levels, called *quantization levels*. The exact value of $f(x,y)$ at the pixel (x,y) is approximated by one of the quantization levels. The more quantization levels are used, the better the approximation is. Usually the highest quantization level is displayed as white, and the lowest as black, and all levels in between are various shades of gray. The quantization levels are the *gray levels*, and they comprise the *gray scale*. Since the gray levels are represented in binary in the computer memory, their number is usually a power of 2. Binary images use 2 gray levels, typical gray scale images are 8-bit, allowing 256 gray levels, but precise, cooled CCD cameras, used in medical applications and astronomy, may produce 10 or 12-bit gray scale images thus allowing 1024 and 4096 gray levels. There are various quantization schemes, uniform, non-uniform, adaptive, that are used to decide what gray levels should be assigned to the pixels, aiming to minimize radiometric distortion.

2.4.5 Image Noise

Undesirable features causing discrepancies in the digital image are considered noise. In microarray image analysis the most damaging noise is background reflection, array misalignment, or scratches and dust on the film surface. Random noise includes the camera noise, as well as random variation in the spot size and shape, *Figure 2-4*. The noise is geometric (spatial discrepancies in the image) or radiometric (discrepancies in the pixel values). The noise sources are external (due to random nature of light, dust in the air, scratches on the objects being observed) or internal (due to the operation of the video sensor itself). The internal noise could be due to the optics, the CCD array[9], [8],[10],[11] or the digitization process[7],[12],[13]. Noise is systematic or random. Systematic noise effects the accuracy of the measurements made from the images, and random noise effects also the precision.

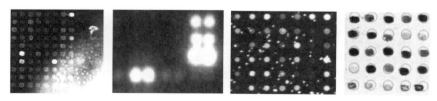

Figure 2-4. Noisy images. From left to right: background illumination, blooming, dust, irregular spots locations and shapes (BioDiscovery, Inc.).

Systematic noise can be minimized by proper use of the sensors, calibration procedures, and proper set up of the experiments. Random noise is always present in the image. It is due to the operation of the electronic equipment and the nature of light itself. Random noise is not reproducible, i.e., there is variability in the pixel values each time images are taken. The use of high quality sensors (scanners and cameras) can reduce the random noise, but it cannot remove it. Although the random noise is not reproducible, it has some general properties that could be characterized using statistical methods. These methods are used to model, detect and estimate the random noise. The goal is to use a noise model, a sensor model, and statistical procedures, so that any inferences that are made from the images are accompanied by quantitative measures of their accuracy and precision. Notice that the systematic and random noise are combined in the image, so treating the systematic noise, by default requires understanding the random noise as well.

2.4.6 Noise Sources

The random noise of the video sensor has three major components: *photon (shot) noise, read noise, and fixed-pattern noise*. The shot noise has external source, it is due to the fluctuations of the photon levels in the incoming light. The read noise is internal. It is related to the physics of the camera and the sensing and measuring process. Major components of read noise are *background noise* and *amplifier noise*. The background noise is due to thermally generated dark current and internal luminance in the camera. Typically, dark current doubles with every increase of 8 degrees Celsius[9]. To reduce dark current cameras are cooled. This is necessary in applications where the signal level is weak compared to the noise level (in astronomy, in some medical applications). In all cases, the background noise is temperature dependent, so cameras must be warmed up before use to allow background noise to stabilize. The non-uniformity in the physical characteristics of the individual sels is manifested in fixed pattern noise in dark images and flat fields. Dark images are images obtained with no presence of light (with lens caps on), flat fields are obtained under uniform illumination (with an integrating sphere or defuse filters). *Impulse noise* is due to pixels whose responses differ significantly from their neighbors. A very high level of impulse noise is manifested as salt and pepper, or speckle noise, and an extremely high over-saturation of pixels, as blooming.

Quantization noise occurs from errors in assigning the pixel gray levels. When the number of quantization levels is not sufficient to represent faithfully the continuous signal, false contours may appear in the digital image. In addition, there is random quantization noise[13]. *Geometric (spatial) noise* is due mainly to the sampling process. The sels spacing puts a limit on the highest spatial frequency that could be recorded in the digital image, and the area of the CCD chip on the lowest one. Geometric distortions in the images are in the center of the digital signal processing literature. In any case, violation of the sampling theorem leads to severe geometric or radiometric distortions,[7],[12]. For high quality digital cameras, these distortions are minimal.

2.5 Color

There are various color models that are used in image processing, most are empirical, and are based on the assumption that a particular color is a mixture of three primary colors. The most popular is the *RGB model*, in which a color, *c*, is represented as a weighted sum of the three primaries, red, green, and blue (R, G, and B),

$$c = rR + gG + bB.$$

The coefficients *r,g,b*, vary between 0 and 1. If we think of the primary colors *R, G, B* as labels on the axes of a coordinate system in a three-dimensional space, all colors that can be represented in this model are points with coordinates (*r,g,b*) and they form a unit cube in three-space, known as the color cube, *Figure 2-5*. In the computer memory color images typically use 8-bits to represent each one of the components, and thus color images are 24-bit.

There are other color models, LUV is used in image compression, CMYK in printing, HSV is perceptually more intuitive for people and is used in computer graphics applications, CYE chromaticity diagram is the empirical model for colors perceived by people[2].

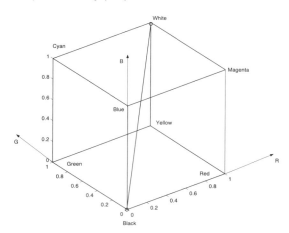

Figure 2-5. A wire frame representation of the color cube. All shades of gray are represented by points on the diagonal from Black(0,0,0) to White(1,1,1). Pure red, green and blue are on the edges from Black to the corresponding Red, Green, and Blue vertices, respectively. The rest of the color points are in the interior, or on the sides.

After introducing the image models and image formation process, we are ready to look at the digital image properties and attributes.

2.6 Digital Image Properties

The image (intensity) histogram is one of the simplest descriptors of digital images. It characterizes globally the image intensity function, $f(x,y)$.

2.6.1 Histogram

The intensity histogram, $h(k)$, of a digital image is a function that counts for each gray level k the number of pixels that have that gray level. Since images have huge number of pixels, $h(k)$ could be very large. For that reason, usually histograms are normalized, i.e., $h(k)$, is divided by the total number of pixels in the image, see Figure 2-6.

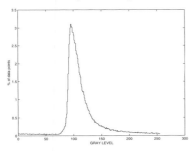 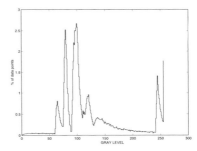

Figure 2-6. Normalized image histograms. The left histogram is on the image on Figure 2-1. The numbers on the vertical axis represent the fraction of pixels that have a particular gray level, 0 to 255.

The histogram shapes in Figure 2-6 exhibit some similarities. Unfortunately similarity in the shapes of the histograms does not imply similarity between the images in general. Two different images might have similar histograms, and still be quite different. For example, two images, showing the same object, in different position and orientation, but on the same background, will have the same histograms (up to variations due to random noise); two binary images with the same numbers of black and white pixels and very different spatial organization of the black and white will have the same histograms as well .

The histogram is used in image enhancement: based on a gray scale transformation called histogram equalization, pixel intensities are changed, so the energy is more uniformly distributed over the gray scale. This enhances the image by brightening darker regions and darkening over saturated with light regions, and thus making features present in those regions more prominent and visible.

The histogram is used often also in intensity, or color, based segmentation which uses the points of local extrema of the histogram to setup thresholds for identifying objects in the images based on the pixel gray levels. The approach might work for clean images, without noise, but the presence of noise makes it impractical. Lets look again at Figure 2-6. The gray levels around the highest peaks of the histograms happen to correspond to the gray level of many of the background pixels in the images. Unfortunately due to noise in the image in *Figure 2-1*, in the left histogram the gray levels around the highest peak cannot be used to classify pixels as background (there are quite a bit of pixels in the foreground that have similar shades to that of the peak, and there are many pixels in the background that differ quite a bit from those). The histogram on the right exhibits another problem, multiple peaks. For that reason, prior to deciding on a threshold for segmentation, images are often subjected to noise suppression algorithms.

Often the term image histogram is used to mean the normalized histogram. The normalized histogram, $\tilde{h}(k)$, is an empirical probability density. If a pixel is selected at random with equal probability from the image, $\tilde{h}(k)$ is the probability that the selected pixel has a gray level k. Related to the normalized histogram is the empirical distribution,

$$\tilde{H}(k) = \sum_{i=0}^{k} \tilde{h}(i).$$

It gives the fraction of pixels in the image with gray level at most k. The empirical distribution may be used in constructing probability models for images treated as stochastic processes.

Next we look at image properties related to the spatial characteristics of the image.

2.6.2. Topological and Metric Properties

Digital images complicate the treatment of distances (*metric*) and neighborhood relations (*topology*) compared to the continuous case. Usually pixels are organized in a rectangular grid. They have finite size and cannot get infinitely small. A neighborhood has to be defined in terms of finite number of close by pixels. From a pixel we can move to another pixel only stepping through grid points.

In case of a rectangular image grid, the most popular topologies are defined by the four- and the eight-nearest neighbors relations. In the *four-nearest neighbors topology*, the neighborhood $U_4(x,y)$ of a pixel (x,y) consist of the pixel itself and its four neighbors, two vertically and two horizontally,

$U_4(x,y) = \{(x,y), (x\text{-}1,y), (x\text{+}1,y), (x,y\text{+}1), (x,y\text{-}1)\}.$

In the *eight-nearest neighbors topology*, the neighborhood $U_8(x,y)$ contains all pixels from $U_4(x,y)$ plus the four closest pixels on diagonal,

$U_8(x,y) = \{(a,b)$ in $U_4(x,y)$, and $(x\text{-}1,y\text{-}1), (x\text{+}1,y\text{-}1), (x\text{-}1,y\text{+}1), (x\text{+}1,y\text{+}1)\}.$

Once a topology is selected, the notions of paths, regions, and a distance are defined. Given two pixels P and Q, a *path* between them is a sequence of pixels $A_1 = P$, $A_2,....,$ $A_{k\text{-}1}$, $A_k = Q$ such that A_i and A_{i+1} are neighbors, for $i = 1,...,k\text{-}1$. In a four-nearest neighbors topology, only horizontal and vertical moves are allowed, and in the eight-nearest neighbors, in addition to horizontal and vertical, also diagonal moves are allowed. The *length of a path* equals the number of pixels in the path minus one, and the *distance* between two pixels is the length of the shortest path connecting them. This definition of a distance for the four-nearest neighbors topology is called "city grid" or "Manhattan" distance, D_4, and for the eight-nearest neighbors topology, the "chessboard" distance, D_8. In terms of pixel coordinates, the formulae for the distance between two points $P(y_1,x_1)$ and $Q(y_2,x_2)$ are given by

$$D_4(P,Q) = |y_2 - y_1| + |x_2 - x_1|,$$

$$D_8(P,Q) = \max(|y_2 - y_1|, |x_2 - x_1|).$$

2.7 Image Features: Edges, Regions, Boundaries

An edge is an image feature, which represents a sharp change in intensity or color. Edges are important because object contours produce edges. An edge has a location specifying where in the image the change occurs, an orientation, specifying the direction in which the change is occurring, and a magnitude giving the strength of the change. Since edges have directions and magnitudes they cannot be represented as scalars, but as vectors fixed at the locations where the changes occur. Technically, the location of an edge (between two pixels) is not part of the digital image, and this creates some complications. In some cases the image is augmented with an additional, edge grid, specifying edge locations[14].

A *region* is a set of pixels any two of which could be connected with a path that is entirely in the set. A region consists of pixels similar with respect to some attribute (for example gray level or color). A complication that arises in the digital domain is that, unlike in the continuous case, in the digital image a closed boundary curve may not separate the image into interior and exterior (background)[4]. Figure 2-7 shows regions and boundaries detected in a part of a microarray image by an image analysis software.

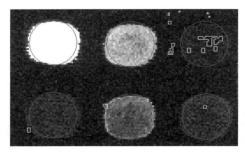

Figure 2-7. A part of a microarray image with extracted region boundaries (BioDiscovery, Inc.)

Next we turn to image operators that are used in detecting image features.

2.8 Spatial Neighborhood Operations: Convolution, Correlation

The convolution and the correlation are one of the most fundamental image processing operations. They are represented as linear systems in the spatial domain. In the discrete case they are, both, defined by a *mask* or *kernel* which is a matrix of relatively small size. The convolution, or a correlation, of an image with a given mask is performed by visiting the image pixels in scan line order. At each visited pixel, first, the mask is centered at the pixel, and then a new value (a coefficient) is calculated using the portion of the image that falls under the mask and the elements of the mask. The resulting matrix of coefficients is the convolution, or correlation, of the image with the mask. The difference between the two operations is that for calculating the convolution the convolution mask is rotated 180 degrees around its center, while the correlation mask is not rotated.

In the context of explaining the convolution and the correlation operators, and spatial filters, a *neighborhood* means the set of close by pixels, where close is defined by the extent of the mask. The result of the convolution and the correlation is another two-dimensional "image" in which the values at the pixels are the calculated coefficients, not the original gray levels. The convolution and the correlation are local operators. This means that the coefficient at a pixel depends only on the gray values in the neighborhood over which the mask extends. The operational differences between a convolution and a correlation are in the way the mask is applied. The application differences are in the problems they address. The convolution's main application is in spatial filtering for detecting spatial features in images, suppressing noise, smoothing. The correlation is used in measuring similarities between images, aligning images, and in detecting image features (objects) by measuring similarity between the image and a template for the feature given by the correlation mask.

2.8.1 Discrete Convolution

The digital convolution, $f * h$, of an image f, of size $M \times N$, with a two-dimensional convolution kernel, h, of size $(2k+1)\times(2k+1)$, is a new two-dimensional array, $g = f * h$, the elements of which are

$$g(x,y) = \sum_{i=-k}^{k} \sum_{j=-k}^{k} f(x\text{-}i,\, y\text{-}j)\, h(i,j).$$

For convenience the indices of the convolution kernel are from $-k$ to k, where k is a small positive number used to define the size of the mask. To keep the range of the convolution result within the gray scale, convolution masks can be normalized, i.e., the elements of the convolution kernel sum to one.

2.8.2 Discrete Correlation

The correlation is defined by

$$g(x,y) = \sum_{i=-k}^{k} \sum_{j=-k}^{k} f(x\text{+}i,\, y\text{+}j)\, h(i,j).$$

Correlation is often used for measuring similarity between images or detecting features. For example, when searching for a feature in a image, a template specifying the feature is defined, then, the correlation of the image with the template is performed. The locations in the correlation image at which highest correlation coefficients are detected are potential feature locations. To account for uniform changes in brightness between images, the correlation coefficients are divided by the total image intensity. Even better approach is to use normalized cross correlation[2].

Next we look at one of the most important application of convolution, *spatial filtering*.

2.9 Spatial Filters

2.9.1 Low-pass Filters: Mean Filters, Gaussian Filters

If all coefficients of the convolution mask are positive, the convolution reduces effectively the high frequencies in the image, i.e. acts as a low-pass filter. If all coefficients are the same and sum to 1, the convolution operation replaces every element with the average of its neighbors. This type of convolution is known as *mean* filter. Mean filters are used in suppression of additive random noise. Larger spatial kernels reduce better noise but also over-smooth the image, i.e., blur edges. More sophisticated are the Gaussian filters. They are circular symmetric convolution masks with positive elements decreasing with distance from the center of the kernel, and approximating a two-dimensional Gaussian (bell shaped surface). A computational advantage in using Gaussian filters is that they are separable, a two dimensional filtering is reduced to the application of two one-dimensional filters.

2.9.2 High-pass filters

Convolution kernels with negative and positive coefficients are designed and act as high-pass filters, enhance edges and contrast. They are used in image enhancement and edge detection.

2.9.3 Rank Filters: Minimum, Maximum, Median

Rank filters are non-linear filters, the coeficients are not wiehgted sums of neighboring pixels. They are based on the order statistics of the neighborhood over which the mask extends. In a rank filtering based on the k-th order statistic, the value of a pixel is replaced by the value of the k-th lowest gray level in its neighborhood. When a pixel value is replaced by the lowest gray level in the neighborhood, the filter is called a *min* filter, when it is replaced with the highest, a *max filter*. The effect of *min* filtering is that the image becomes darker, and of *max* filtering brighter, but in both cases non-linear blurring results. *Min* and *max* filters usually are used as steps in image analysis procedures, not as stand alone ones. When a pixel value is replaced by the median gray level in the neighborhood the filter is called a *median filter*. The median filter does not have a tendency to over-smooth as the mean filters. It is useful in removing impulse noise where the number of noisy pixels is at most half the number of all pixels in the neighborhood. The disadvantage is that the median filter can also remove image detail appearing in less than half of the neighborhood. In an attempt to combine the advantages of both the mean and the median filters, and to remedy the sensitivity of the mean to extreme, noisy, data, α-trimmed mean filters are designed.

2.9.4 Mixture Filters

The α-*trimmed mean* filters are examples of mixtures of non-linear and linear filters. First ranking in the neighborhood is conducted, extreme values are trimmed, and then the mean of the rest of the values is taken to replace the pixel at the center of the neighborhood. The value α specifies how many pixel values should be trimmed at each end. When α is zero, the α-trimmed mean filter is a mean filter; when α is $((2k+1)^2 -1)/2$, the α-trimmed mean filter is a median filter. Here the kernel (mask) is of size $(2k+1)$ x $(2k+1)$. α-trimmed mean filters perform better than mean and median filters when both types, additive and impulse noise are present. This is still not the end of the story. The problem is that image noise may vary spatially, and thus choosing "one filter fits all" strategy might be too restrictive.

2.9.5 Adaptive Filters

In *adaptive filtering*, the filter is selected based on the properties of the local neighborhood. Adaptive filters are appropriate when the noise characteristics vary spatially, and a single filter does not perform well on the whole image. An example of an adaptive filter is the minimum mean square error (MMSE) filter[5]. MMSE filter acts as a mean filter in relatively homogeneous intensity regions, and suppresses noise in those regions, but in regions with edges, it does not smooth the edges, but also it does not reduce the noise.

2.9.6 Liner Filtering in the Frequency-Domain

From the duality of the spatial- and frequency-domain representations of the linear shift-invariant systems, it follows that there are two approaches to filtering that use frequency-domain representations. One is based on the *convolution theorem*: use computations in the frequency domain to carry out filtering for an already designed spatial filter. First pad the kernel with zeros, so that the image and the kernel have the same size, next compute the Fourier transforms of the image and the zero-padded kernel, then multiplying the two Fourier transforms, and last compute the inverse Fourier transform of that product. Although it seems that there is quite a bit of computations to be preformed, all of the above calculations on big images in the frequency-domain are more efficient than the computation of the convolution in the spatial domain. The other approach, which is most often used, is to design the filter directly in the frequency-domain by constructing the transfer function of the linear system.

Finally, we are ready to turn our attention to image quality and noise.

2.10 Image Quality and Parameter Estimation in the Presence of Noise

As described earlier, there are various sources of noise in the digital image. The noise poses a problem for inferences of quantitative measurements from the images. One way to resolve the problem is to preprocess the images, to remove or suppress the noise, i.e., do image restoration, or cleaning. The other is to use statistical inference procedures that can deal with random noise in the images.

We already discussed the use of spatial filters in noise suppression. Here we turn to stochastic approaches which make inferences in the presence of noise. They include several ingredients: a sensor (sample) model, a noise model, and possibly a prior model.

Let **X** represents the original undistorted unobservable image. The observed image **Z** is obtained from **X** through some degradation transformation Ψ, thus the *sensor* model is

$$Z = \Psi(X, \varepsilon)$$

where ε is a random field modeling the noise process. Good sensor models are hard to build. In practice simplifications are made. The simplest is the *location data model*,

$$Z = X + \varepsilon.$$

Popular is the *linear model* with additive noise,

$$Z = H(X) + \varepsilon.$$

Here H is linear spatial filter, modeling image degradation, which is independent of the noise. One such degradation is an image blur due to the optics of the video sensor.

The general noise model assumes that the image noise ε is a sum of image-dependent random noise and image-independent random noise components[1]. For every pixel (x, y), the noise at the pixel is modeled by

$$\varepsilon_{xy} = g(x, y)\alpha_{xy} + \beta_{xy},$$

where α and β are random fields, and g is a spatial function, and the indices x, y are used to index the individual components of the random fields, and to refer to the value of g at the pixel. By varying the distributions models of α and β, and the form of g, this general noise model is used to characterize various noise sources and types of image noise[1]. In many applications, the noise components are assumed independent. Often they are represented as white noise. A special case of a white noise is Gaussian white noise, which is characterized by its mean and covariance functions, and by the finite joint distributions.

The additive noise model has lead to the definition of the term signal to noise ratio, which is used to characterize video sensors and noise levels in images.

2.10.1 Signal to Noise Ratio

The signal to noise ratio is defined as the ratio of mean signal to mean error,

$$SNR = \frac{E[Z]}{E[\varepsilon]}$$

Good images have high signal to noise ratios. Sensor signal to noise ratios are reported by sensor manufacturers, and this parameter should be considered when selecting the sensors.

Statistical methods are used to estimate the true unobserved image attributes, from the observed images, given the noise model. In order to make a statistical inference, some criteria for optimality must be selected. We briefly present some results from estimation theory that are most often used in image analysis. To simplify the notation, we use the one-dimensional case, i.e. we use random variables, not random fields. Definitions related to random variables and probability theory are given in the Supplement 2A.

2.10.2 Estimation

Let Z be a random variable being observed, and it is desired to estimate the value of a random variable X, provided a sensor model.

The *minimum mean square error* (**MMSE**) method searches for an estimate, $\theta = \hat{X}$, of X that minimize the mean square error function

$$s(\theta) = E[(X - \theta)^2].$$

Given an observation, z, the mean square estimate is the conditional mean, $E[(X \mid z)]$.

In case of images, *Wiener filtering* is an image restoration method, which uses a sensor model with blurring function and additive noise, and it produces the optimal estimate in terms of MMSE,[1].

Bayesian estimation includes, in addition to sensor and noise models, a *prior* probability model for the unobservable, true image (parameter). The *maximum a posteriori estimate* (**MAP**) maximizes the posterior distribution, i.e. it is close to the observed data, and it is faithful to the characteristics modeled by the prior. A more sophisticated *Bayes inference* method is to incorporate explicitly a *loss function* in addition to the sensor model, the noise model, and the prior. The loss function quantifies the penalties that must be paid depending how far the estimate is from the true unobserved value. Optimal estimates in this case are produced by computational procedures called *Bayes rules*. *Robust statistical estimation* methods produce quality estimates even when the actual data deviate from the modeling assumptions.

2.11 Further Reading

With this we conclude the introductory chapter to image analysis. The exposition is not complete, and it cannot be within the limited space we have here. For in depth treatment of image analysis methods the reader is referred to books in digital image processing. The text by Gonzalez and Woods[2], is the classical textbook for readers with good mathematical background. The book, by Jain[1], although not very new, is a very thorough textbook at a graduate level. An excellent, and up to date reference is the "Handbook of Video and Image Processing"[3]. It requires mathematical background at an undergraduate level. Slonka et al.[4], ties up nicely together image processing and computer vision techniques. The intended audience is engineers. For very accessible treatment of image processing topics, for readers without extensive mathematics background, we recommend the book by Efford[5]. Although Efford's book is targeted to readers interested in programming, the problems are explained clearly, and the programming details could be skipped without hampering the exposition.

SUPPLEMENT 2A

Mathematical Foundations of Image Analysis

The Fourier Transform

Next we give the definition and summarize the properties of the Fourier transform of continuous functions, and then we give the discrete versions for digital images. For more in depth treatment we refer the reader to[2,3].

Given a continuous, integrable function $f(x,y)$ of two independent variables x and y, its *Fourier transform*, $F(u,v)$, is the complex-valued function of two independent variables u and v, defined by

$$F(u,v) = \int_{-\infty}^{\infty} \int_{-\infty}^{\infty} f(x,y)\exp[-j2\pi(ux + vy)]dxdy,$$

where j is the imaginary unit defined by $j = \sqrt{-1}$. Given $F(u,v)$, $f(x,y)$ can be obtained by the *inverse Fourier transform*,

$$f(x,y) = \int_{-\infty}^{\infty} \int_{-\infty}^{\infty} F(u,v)\exp[j2\pi(ux + vy)]dudv.$$

The functions $f(x,y)$ and $F(u,v)$ are called a *Fourier transform pair*. The pair is unique, i.e. either function from the pair can be obtained from the other using the forward or the inverse Fourier transform, and both transformations model exactly the same image.

The Fourier transform pair in one-dimension is defined by the equations

$$F(u) = \int_{-\infty}^{\infty} f(x)\exp[-j2\pi xu]dx, \quad f(x) = \int_{-\infty}^{\infty} F(u)\exp[j2\pi xu]du.$$

The Convolution Operator

If $h(x,y)$ and $f(x,y)$ are two-dimensional continuous functions, their *convolution*, g, denoted by $g = h*f = f*h$, is defined by

$$g(x,y) = \int_{-\infty}^{\infty} \int_{-\infty}^{\infty} f(a,b)h(x-a,y-b)dadb = \int_{-\infty}^{\infty} \int_{-\infty}^{\infty} f(x-a,y-b)h(a,b)dadb$$

In the discrete case the integrals are replaced by summations, and $h(x,y)$ is usually a square array of relatively small size. It is a linear spatial filter. We discussed in more detail the discrete convolution and its application in the chapter.

The *convolution theorem* states the duality between convolution in the spatial-domain and multiplication of the frequency-domain, and it is expressed in the Convolution/Multiplication properties in Table 2-1.

Properties of the Fourier Transform

In the spatial-domain $f(x,y)$ is an intensity function, and x and y represent spatial coordinates. In the frequency-domain, u and v are spatial frequencies that represent intensity changes with respect to spatial distances[1]. The units of u and v are reciprocal to those of x and y, respectively. The two-dimensional Fourier transform can be computed by computing successfully two one-dimensional Fourier transforms with respect to x and y separately,

$$F(u,v) = \int_{-\infty}^{\infty} \left[\int_{-\infty}^{\infty} f(x,y)\exp[-j2\pi ux]dx \right] \exp[-j2\pi vy]dy.$$

In particular, when $f(x,y)$ is separable, i.e., $f(x,y) = f_1(x)f_2(y)$, the above equation implies that $F(u,v)$ is also separable (see separability property in the table).

Properties of the two-dimensional Fourier transform are summarized in Table 2-1[1]. In the table, f_i and $F_i, i = 1,2$, are Fourier transform pairs, and so are h and H, and g and G; $\bar{f}(x,y)$ denotes the complex conjugate of $f(x,y)$. Since images are represented by real-valued functions, by the symmetric property it follows that the Fourier transform of an image has a conjugate symmetry.

The rotational property of the Fourier transform pair is expressed as follows. If an image is rotated around the origin by an angle θ, the Fourier transform of the rotated image is exactly the Fourier transform of the original image rotated by the same angle θ. In particular, if θ is 180 degrees, i.e., the rotation is a reflection, we obtain that $f(-x,-y)$ and $F(-x,-y)$ are a Fourier transform pair.

Notice that $F(u,v)$ is a complex-valued function

$$F(u,v) = R(u,v) + jI(u,v),$$

Table 2-1. Properties of the Fourier transform

Property name	Function $f(x,y)$	Fourier transform $F(u,v)$
Conjugtion	$\bar{f}(x,y)$	$\bar{F}(-u,-v)$
Linearity	$a_1 f_1(x,y) + a_2 f_2(x,y)$	$a_1 F_1(u,v) + a_2 F_2(u,v)$
Separability	$f_1(x) f_2(y)$	$F_1(u) F_2(v)$
Scaling	$f(ax, by)$	$(\lvert ab \rvert)^{-1} F(u/a, v/b)$
Shifting	$f(x-x_0, y-y_0)$	$\exp[-j2\pi(x_0 u + y_0 v)] F(x,y)$
Modulation	$\exp[j2\pi(u_0 x + v_0 y)] f(x,y)$	$F(u-u_0, v-v_0)$
Convolution	$g(x,y) = h(x,y) * f(x,y)$	$G(u,v) = H(u,v) F(u,v)$
Multiplication	$g(x,y) = h(x,y) f(x,y)$	$G(u,v) = H(u,v) * F(u,v)$
Symmetry	$\bar{f}(x,y) = f(x,y)$	$\bar{F}(u,v) = F(-u,-v)$

with real and imaginary parts $R(u,v)$ and $I(u,v)$, respectively. Complex values can be expressed in another form, using a magnitude and a phase angle

$$F(u,v) = \lvert F(u,v) \rvert \exp[j\phi(u,v)],$$

$$\lvert F(u,v) \rvert = \sqrt{R(u,v)^2 + I(u,v)^2}$$

$$\theta(u,v) = arctan \frac{I(u,v)}{R(u,v)}$$

The functions $\lvert F(u,v) \rvert$, $\phi(u,v)$, and $\lvert F(u,v) \rvert^2$ are called *Fourier magnitude (amplitude), phase, and power spectra* of $f(x,y)$, respectively.

The Discrete Fourier Transform

The Fourier transform of a digital image always exists. For technical reasons the digital image is extended periodically to infinity, i.e., instead the original limited rectangular image area, the extended image consists of infinitely many replicated copies of the original that tile an infinite two-dimensional grid. For a digital image $f(x,y)$ of size $M \times N$, the extension is defined by $f(x+kM,y+lN)=f(x,y)$, where $x = 0,1,...,M-1$, $y = 0,1,...,N-1$, and k,l are integers. Although the extended image is infinite, since it is periodic, only finite number of samples, $f(x,y)$, can be used to represent it. The Fourier transform of the original image is, by definition, the Fourier transform of the extended image. It is periodic with a period M in the first independent variable, and N in the second one. For a digital image $f(x,y)$ of size $M \times N$, the forward *discrete Fourier transform* is given by

$$F(u,v) = \frac{1}{MN}\sum_{x=0}^{M-1}\sum_{y=0}^{N-1} f(x,y)\exp\left[-j2\pi\left(\frac{ux}{M} + \frac{vy}{N}\right)\right]$$

$$u = 0,1,...,M-1, \quad v = 0,1,...,N-1$$

If the image grid have separations Δx and Δy, the grid on which $F(u,v)$ is specified is spaced by Δu and Δv, respectively, where

$$\Delta u = \frac{1}{M\Delta x} \qquad \Delta v = \frac{1}{N\Delta y}$$

Using the *inverse discrete Fourier transform*, $f(x,y)$ is expressed as a weighted sum of complex exponentials with coefficients $F(u,v)$,

$$f(x,y) = \sum_{u=0}^{M-1}\sum_{v=0}^{N-1} F(u,v)\exp\left[j2\pi\left(\frac{ux}{M} + \frac{vy}{N}\right)\right]$$

$$x = 0,1,...,M-1, \quad y = 0,1,...,N-1$$

The magnitude, phase, and power spectra of the discrete Fourier transform are defined the same way as in the continuous case. The so called **DC** coefficient, $F(0,0)$, is the average intensity over the whole image. Each coefficient, $F(u,v)$, of the Fourier transform of an image carries information about the sinusoidal changes of particular frequencies u and v over the whole image. The nature of natural images is such that lower spatial frequency components of the signal have higher energy than the high frequency components. Thus, the magnitudes of the coefficients with frequencies u and v that are closer to zero are larger than the magnitudes of coefficients corresponding to higher frequencies. The low-frequency coefficients concentrate most of the energy. See Figure 2-8, which shows an amplitude (magnitude) spectrum as an image. The (0,0), frequency location is at the center of the image. The bright spot in the center of the image represents the magnitude of the DC coefficient. Darker regions correspond to coefficients with smaller magnitudes. The symmetry of the Fourier spectrum is clearly expressed in the image.

By the Euler's formula,

$$\exp[j\theta] = \cos\theta + j\sin\theta,$$

if we substitute the exponentials in the expression for $f(x,y)$ above, with the sum of the corresponding sine and cosine functions, we obtain $f(x,y)$ as a weighted sum of basis two-dimensional sinusoidal functions. The weights are given by the Fourier coefficients $F(u,v)$. A two-dimensional sinusoidal wave is characterized by its amplitude, its phase shift, and also its orientation (direction of propagation). A sinusoidal function that is restricted to a finite image domain has a frequency, which is measured in cycles per pixel or cycles per image. The Fourier coefficient $F(u,v)$ is nonzero if the image contains intensity pattern that is a two-dimensional sinusoid of frequencies u and v. The magnitude and phase spectra specify the amplitude and phase shift of the corresponding sinusoidal waves. The representations of the images in the spatial-domain, via $f(x,y)$, or in the frequency-domain, via $F(u,v)$, are equivalent, in the sense that they specify the same image, and going from one representation to the other by the Fourier transform and its inverse does not lead to any loss of information or distortion. The Fourier spectrum, $|F(u,v)|$, is sensitive to the strength and orientation of certain features present in the image, but it does not encode any location information. The location information is encoded by the phase spectrum, $\phi(u,v)$. If the Fourier amplitude spectrum is degraded, the relative brightness of features in the image cannot be recovered faithfully, but if the phase spectrum is degraded, the spatial coherence of the image is degraded, and features are lost. For that reason, most image processing techniques when using the Fourier transform manipulate the amplitude, but not the phase,[5].

Displaying the Fourier Transform

The Fourier transform of an image is a complex valued function, so it cannot be displayed as an image. Usually, the real-valued Fourier magnitude (amplitude) spectrum is displayed. There is a slight problem though. The amplitude spectrum has a range much wider than the dynamic range of a typical display hardware. To enhance the display of the Fourier spectrum as an image, a useful technique is to use a logarithm function and compress the range of the spectrum first. The function that is suitable for display is

$$D(u,v) = c\log[1+|F(u,v)|],$$

here c is a chosen positive constant. Another issue is related to the symmetry and the periodicity of the discrete Fourier transform. The symmetry is with respect to the origin. The origin of an image traditionally is at the top-left (bottom-left) corner. To exemplify the symmetry in the Fourier spectrum, it is more natural to display the center of symmetry at the center of the image, thus moving the **DC** coefficient to the center. For an image of size M x N this means shifting the origin at the center with coordinates $(M/2, N/2)$. By the modulation property, the shift of the origin in the frequency domain can be carried out by multiplication with a complex exponential in the spatial-domain. For square images, this complex exponential is simply $(-1)^{(x+y)}$. In Figure 2-8 we have used these techniques to display the Fourier magnitude spectrum for the image in Figure 2-1.

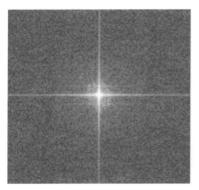

Figure 2-8. The Fourier amplitude spectrum, $|F(u,v)|$, of the image represented in Figure 2-1. The DC coefficient is displayed at the center of the image.

Definitions and Results from Probability Theory

We use the following notation: random variables are denoted with upper case letter, and particular observations of them (samples), with lower case.

A random variable is specified by its cumulative distribution functions. For a real-valued random variable, Z, *the distribution* is defined by

$$F_Z(z) = P[Z \leq z],$$

where $P[Z \leq z]$ is the probability of the event that the value of the random variable Z is less than or equal to z. A continuous random variable can be specified also by its probability *density* function,

$$f_Z(z)dz = P[z < Z \le z + dz],$$

where $P[z < Z \le z + dz]$ denotes the probability of the event that the value of the random variable Z is within the interval $(z, z + dz)$, and dz denotes an infinitely small increment. And if the distribution function is differentiable, the density is its derivative,

$$f_Z(z) = \frac{dF}{dz}(z)$$

A discrete random variable is specified by its *point mass function* (pmf), confusingly also often called density function, or by its distribution

$$f_Z(z) = P[Z = z], \quad F_Z(z) = \sum_x fZ(x),$$

where the summation is taken over all values $x, x \le z$. The expected value (mean, or first moment), $E[Z]$ of a random variable is defined by

$$E[Z] = \int_{-\infty}^{\infty} z dF_Z(z)$$

In case of discrete random variables the mean is simply the average weighted according to the point mass function

$$E[Z] = \sum z f_Z(z).$$

where the sum is taken over all possible values of Z. The variance (also called second centered moment) of a random variable is defined by

$$Var[Z] = E[(Z - EZ)^2] = E[Z^2] - (E[Z])^2$$

It characterizes the variability of the random variable around the mean. The expected value, $E[Z^2]$, is called second moment (this should clarify the name for the variance - second centered moment). Given two random variables X and Y their covariance is defined by

$$Cov[X,Y] = E[(X - E[X])(Y - E[Y])] = E[XY - E[X]E[Y]].$$

In image processing we work with random fields, which are collections of random variables. Thus it is desirable to know how random variables relate to each other, and if some information about one of them could be gained from the properties and the observations of the rest, or in another context, if properties of an ideal, unobservable image can be inferred from an observed sample of a random field. In discussing such relations and making such inferences, the notions of independence, conditional density, and conditional expectation are of great importance. We give their definitions next.

Let X and Y be two random variables, the *joint distribution* $F_{XY}(x,y)$ is the probability of the event that $X \leq x$ and $Y \leq y$,

$$F_{XY}(x,y) = P\,[X \leq x, Y \leq y],$$

and the *joint density* is defined similarly,

$$f_{XY}(x,y)dxdy = P\,[x < X \leq x+dx,\ y < Y \leq y+dy].$$

The two random variables are *independent* if their joint density (distribution) is simply the product of their individual densities (distributions),

$$f_{XY}(x,y) = f_X(x)f_Y(y).$$

The correlation of independent random variables is zero, but only for normally distributed random variables (with Gaussian distributions) uncoreleated, implies independent.

The conditional density of X given Y, denoted by $f_{X\mid Y}(x\mid y)$ is defined by

$$f_{X\mid Y}(x\mid y) = \frac{f_{XY}(x,y)}{f_Y(y)}\ .$$

If X and Y are independent, $f_{X\mid Y}(x\mid y)=f_X(x)$, in a sense, knowledge about the value of Y does not change the information about the value of X.

The conditional expectation, $E[X\mid y]$, is the expected value of X with respect to the conditional density, where y is an observation of Y,

$$E[X\mid y] = \int_{-\infty}^{\infty} x f_{X\mid Y}(x\mid y)dx$$

Note that as a function of the random variable of Y, the conditional expectation, $E[X\mid Y]$ is a random variable.

To the study of stochastic processes of interest are the marginal distributions and densities of the process which characterize the behavior of a subset of random variables from the collection when the values of the rest of the variables in the collection is fixed.

A Gaussian (normal) distribution is completely specified by its mean μ and variance σ^2. A one-dimensional Gaussian distribution, $N(\mu,\sigma)$, with parameters μ and σ has a probability density function

$$f(x|\mu,\sigma) = \frac{1}{\sqrt{2\pi\sigma^2}} \int_{-\infty}^{\infty} \exp\left[-\frac{1}{2}\left(\frac{x-\mu}{\sigma}\right)^2\right]$$

The standard normal distribution, $N(0,1)$, has mean 0 and variance 1. The multivariate Gaussian distribution is parametrized by its mean and covariance matrices.

A random field Z is specified by its *joint distribution function*,

$$F_Z(z) = P[Z_{xy} \le z_{xy} : x = 0,1,...M\text{-}1, y = 0,1,...N\text{-}1]$$

where z is the collection of z_{xy} values over all pixel sites, and

$$P[Z_{xy} \le z_{xy} : x = 0,1,...M\text{-}1, y = 0,1,...N\text{-}1]$$

denotes the probability of the joint event that the values of $Z_{xy} \le z_{xy}$, for every pixel site (x,y).

References

1. *Jain A*: Fundamentals of Digital Image Processing, *Upper Saddle River, Prentice-Hall,* 1989.

2. *Gonzalez R, Woods R*: Digital Image Processing, *Addison-Wesley Publishing Company,* 2nd ed. 2002.

3. *Bovik A* (Ed.): Handbook of Image and Video Processing, *Academic Press*, 2000.

4. *Slonka M, Hlavac V, Boyle R*: Image Processing, Analysis, and Machine Vision, 2nd. Ed., *Brooks/Cole Publishing Company*, 1999.

5. *Efford N*: Digital Image Processing a Practical Introduction Using Java, *Pearson Education Limited*, 2000.

6. *Ripley BD*: Statistical Inference for Spatial Processes, *Cambridge University Press,* 1988.

7. *Lenz R, Fritsch D*: Accuracy of Videometry with CCD Sensors. *AISPRS Journal of Photogrammetry and Remote Sensing* 1990; 45:90-110.

8. *Theuwissen A*: Solid-state Imaging with Charge Coupled Devices, *Kluwer Academic Publishers*, 1995.

9. *Baynon E, Lamb D*: Charged-coupled Devices and their Application, *McGraw-Hill,* 1980.

10. *Holst G*: CCD Arrays, Cameras, and Displays, Winter Park, FL:*JCD Pub*. 1996.

11. *Snyder D,et al.*: Compensation for Readout Noise in CCD Image. *Journal of Optical Society of America* 1995; 12(2):272-283.

12 *Beyer H*: Linejitter and Geometric Calibration of CCD Cameras. *ISPRS Journal of Photogrammetry and Remote Sensing* 1990; 45:17-32.

13. *Sripad A, Snyder D*: A necessary and Sufficient Condition for the Quantization Noise to be Uniform and White. IEEE Trans. *On Acoustic, Speech, and Signal Processing* 1977, AASP-25(5):442-448.

14. *Geman S, Geman D*: Stochastic Relaxation, Gibbs Distribution, and the Bayesian Restoration of Images. *IEEE Trans. on Pattern Analysis and Machine Intelligence* 1984; 6(6):721-741.

ADVANTAGES OF LASER CONFOCAL MICROARRAY SCANNING

Mark McGovern, Ph.D. *and* Reda Fayek, Ph.D.

Contact:

Virtek Biotechnology, 785 Bridge Street, Waterloo, Ontario Canada N2V 2K1
E-mail: markmcgovernphd@hotmail.com   reda.fayek@IEEE.org

0-9664027-5-8/02/$0.00+$.50   *From:* **Microarray Image Analysis-Nuts & Bolts** (pp.51-68)
©2002 by DNA Press, LLC   Edited by: S. Shah and G. Kamberova

3.1 Introduction

Microarray technology has progressed rapidly over the past year, evolving from mainly a qualitative, first look at gene expression, to a more quantitative and scientific approach to generating biological data. Biochips are advancing beyond genomic research into the areas of proteomics and diagnostic uses. Biology researchers are becoming more aware of the different approaches and technologies used in printing, scanning, image analysis and data mining. This can be overwhelming given the number of different components, manufacturers, and strategies that exist today. Although the industry has not yet standardized to any one paradigm, microarray technology continues to evolve towards becoming a reliable, reproducible scientific tool for biology.

The purpose of this chapter is to provide a general understanding of the different approaches used to design commercial microarray scanners. Particular attention is given to laser confocal microarray scanners, as they have particular advantages.

3.2 Microarrays and Scanning - Features and Parameters

A wide variety of scanners for microarray analysis exist on the market today. They differ in many respects: technology, size, speed, sensitivity, capacity and many more. Attempting to make wide-sweeping generalizations about which type of scanner is better than another, or how microarray experiments should be done, is a daunting task because the field of biochip microarrays is quickly evolving. The following discussion provides an overview of many key points of interest concerning microarray scanners and the different points of view concerning their design.

3.2.1 Resolution

Microarray scanners need to be flexible enough to accommodate future needs. A good example of this relates to the size of the human genome and how it impacts on DNA microarrays. Prior to the year 2000, it was widely believed that the human genome contained roughly 100,000 genes. To construct a microarray on a standard microscope slide containing the entire human genome, every feature on the chip would need to measure no more than about 30 microns in diameter. A frequently-used rule of thumb is that the scanning resolution of each pixel should be set at 1/10 the diameter of the spot being scanned. In our case, this would be a pixel resolution of about 3 microns. This implies that the scanner must be built to a specification that allowed it to accurately scan an entire microscope slide at 3 μm resolution, a daunting task, but one that has been accomplished. However, when the first draft of the human genome was announced in mid-2000, the biology universe changed, and then the number of genes in the human genome was postulated to number between

30,000 and 40,000 genes. Since fewer spots were needed, the 3μm resolution was no longer necessary because the spots could be made larger - or so it seemed. However, microarray users are finding that having only one copy of each gene feature per chip may not be sufficient to generate reliable data. In order to calculate statistics, such as confidence intervals, it is necessary to include replicates, positive and negative controls, and introduce quality control features. So, in theory, a well-designed complete human genome microarray chip could still contain 100,000 features, many of which being replicates and controls. Whether such a chip will be made in significant numbers and adopted by users remains to be seen.

3.2.2 Sensitivity

Another critical feature of microarray scanners is their sensitivity. Generating a "good" image from microarray scanners can be challenging because the quantity of fluorescently-labeled DNA hybridized to the probes on the microarray is not very large. Additionally, the glass substrate for the microarray generates a low, but significant, level of background fluorescence. Therefore, it is necessary to use extremely sensitive scanning and detection strategies that enable the scanner to detect the faint signals and block out as much of the undesirable background fluorescence as possible. Such strategies should exploit the complex relations between the fluorophore concentrations in the spots, the excitation source characteristics and the detection mechanism and its properties. A simple way to increase sensitivity is to increase the power of the excitation light source in an attempt to make the fluorophores emit greater quantities of fluorescent light. However, it is known that organic fluorophores can only be excited a finite number of times before they are photobleached, which means the dye undergoes a permanent chemical change and is destroyed. The topic of photobleaching will be addressed further in the discussion on light sources. It is also possible to increase sensitivity by increasing the detector gain (often referred to as detector sensitivity). Depending on the type of detector, there usually is an optimal setting for detector gain, and increasing the gain further often results in increased noise which is unwanted. Therefore, diminishing returns are encountered when attempts are made to increase sensitivity by increasing the power of the light source or increasing detector gain beyond certain limits. However, if the optimal combination of components is chosen, then excellent sensitivity can be achieved.

3.2.3. Multiple Dyes

It is difficult to control the quantity of gene probe material deposited into each feature on the DNA microarray. It is also challenging to evenly hybridize the sample across the entire microarray. Therefore, a control sample should be mixed in with the experimental sample to act as an internal standard. The control sample and experimental sample should be each labeled with a different dye, and ultimately, the ratio of the fluorophore intensities is used as a measure of gene up- or down-regulation. Therefore, the absorption and emission spectral curves of the two dyes must be well separated to minimize cross-talk. Cross-talk results from either the simultaneous excitation of multiple dyes by one light source, the simultaneous detection of multiple dyes in one detector channel, or both. Some microarray users wish to incorporate more than two dyes into one experiment, perhaps to add additional controls, or to generate more data from one slide. The risk of cross-talk increases as the number of dyes used increases, because most organic fluorophores have rather broad absorption and emission spectral curves. Cross-talk can be reduced by selecting filters that have a narrow spectral range, at the expense of reduced sensitivity.

3.2.4 Microarray Substrates

The substrate is the material on which the DNA probe will be printed. With the increase in the number of applications, many different types of microarray substrates became available. Besides the well-known glass substrate, it is possible to use gold-plated, silicon, plastic or membrane-coated materials. Substrates which have wells engraved into their surfaces can be used for "wet" applications. The reasons for choosing a specific type of substrate are varied. Some users may want to experiment with different adhesion chemistries that are only available on these different materials. Other users may want to eliminate background fluorescence that is commonly seen in glass slides. Still other users may want to detect biological molecules dissolved in buffered solution, perhaps to detect enzymatic activity or observe protein-protein interactions. Often benefits of using new substrate materials come with trade-offs. Many of these materials are highly reflective, and will direct the excitation light back into the detection optics and reduce the signal-to-background ratio, unless the scanner uses the proper optical design. Wells often have reflective walls and bottoms, and the biological materials of interest may be present at the bottom of the wells, or in the bulk solution. Coverslips present an interface where multiple reflections can occur. Some provision for reducing reflections and the ability to scan into wells or beneath coverslips should be considered.

3.2.5 Speed

It is desirable to scan a microarray as fast as possible. However, there is a trade-off between several variables. Increasing scan resolution and/or scan area usually decreases the scanning speed if the same level of sensitivity is required. This is because the scanner must "dwell" over each pixel for a certain amount of time to collect enough light for a valid signal to be reported, and increasing the number of pixels will lengthen the amount of time needed to generate the image. Scanning multiple dyes simultaneously will increase the scan speed, but increases the risk of cross-talk.

3.2.6 Ease of Use

The number of steps required to operate the instrument and scan a microarray should be minimal to allow a greater number of users to run their experiments under minimal supervision. An intuitive graphical user interface is essential. However, if the scanner's graphical user interface (GUI) is too simple, it is no longer flexible to utilize different scanning protocols and adjust the parameters to maximize data quality. For the uncritical user, an oversimplified GUI may suggest that the first image seen on the monitor screen is the best one the instrument could produce.

3.2.7 High Quality Data

Above all, the quality of the image generated by the microarray scanner must satisfy certain criteria for producing valid data. For instance the signal-to-noise ratios of the spot should be sufficiently high so automatic spot finding algorithms can readily detect the spot signal from its surrounding background signal. Equally important is that each pixel value is accurately registered. This means that each data pixel directly corresponds with the actual feature on the microarray that is being imaged. The resolution of the scanner must be sufficiently high to provide enough pixels per spot for image analysis algorithms to accurately analyze the spot intensities. Misregistered pixels, especially around the edges of the spot, can lead to difficulties in defining the spot location, shape, and size, which will impact the spot intensity calculations. Of course, there are other causes of low quality data, and errors can occur during the manufacture of the microarrays, the fluorescent labeling protocols, and during hybridization. A "systems analyst" approach of looking at all of the components of the entire microarray process is often a superior way to improve the ultimate data quality, rather than focusing on just one part of the process such as the scanner.

Due to the above mentioned factors, it can be seen that there are many contradicting demands on the design of a microarray scanner, and that all of these factors interact with one another. Some of these factors are: sensitivity, resolution, multiple types of dyes and substrates, speed, and ease of use. Above all, the ultimate goal of the microarray scanner is to produce high-quality data.

3.3 Basic Scanner Components

Microarray scanners have quickly evolved into very complex instruments involving not only the optical package, but also sophisticated software and automation. Nevertheless, all scanners require the following components:

- Light source(s) to activate the fluorescent molecules present on the array surface.

- A strategy for exciting the fluorophores in a way that maximizes utility and minimizes undesired effects.

- The optical design that provides a means of scanning the sample at the desired resolution.

- Detector(s) for measuring the magnitude of the fluorescence signals.

- A mechanism for orienting the slide and positioning during scanning.

3.4 Light Sources

A scanner can use a white light source, or a laser light source (*Table 3-1*). White light sources usually are based on the output of a Xenon lamp or similar source that generates light with wavelengths from about 350nm to 750nm or more. Filters are used to select the desired wavelength range. White light sources have the advantage of a single source that generates multiple excitations selectable by the user. Laser light sources are not as flexible since they have fixed wavelengths. However, white light sources are typically large in size and generate a large quantity of heat.

Many scanners use laser light sources to excite fluorescently-labeled biomolecules present on the array surface. There are two basic categories; gas lasers and solid-state lasers. Gas lasers, commonly used in scientific instruments, have certain disadvantages. As the name suggests, a gas laser is essentially a tube filled with a certain gas which is used as the lasing medium. They tend to be large and occupy valuable bench-space, and their power output usually drops significantly over the operational life of the gas laser. A half-life time (time before the power output drops to 50% of maximum) of about 10,000 hours is typical. Gas lasers also tend to produce large amounts of heat, both from the gas tube and from the power supply. Running a gas laser without providing a means of cooling the laser will usually result in a much shorter laser lifespan. Finally, the gas laser must be "warmed up" for at least 15 minutes before use, and during use, it cannot be "gated" or quickly turned on and off during scanning. The gas laser must be left on during the entire scanning session, which will effectively shorten its lifespan while it is idling, relative to a laser that can be gated on and off as required.

In contrast, a solid-state laser is usually much smaller in size, and is more efficient in terms of minimizing heat production. Unlike gas lasers with fixed power, a critical advantage of solid-state lasers is that their intensity can be controlled with closed loop feedback mechanisms. Another major advantage is the ability to gate the laser during scanning. Since most laser scanners use at least two lasers, but only one laser is needed to excite one fluorophore at a time, gating effectively doubles the lifetime of the solid state laser because it is only turned on when it is needed. A non-gated scanner must use a shutter, or some means of blocking out one of the lasers when it is not required, and therefore, its energy is being wasted. Virtek's expertise in manufacturing laser systems has been applied in laser marking, quality control and other applications in diverse industries. In these settings, the lasers are run under much harsher conditions than found in a laser scanner intended for biology applications. For example, a roof truss factory employing a laser marking system typically has high levels of temperature and humidity. Some units have been in the field for more than 5 years, and the laser diodes have not shown any significant level of aging in any installation. Much of this success is due to paying particular attention to monitoring the laser power output with a feedback circuit, and using the minimum power necessary to achieve the objective to extend the laser life.

Table 3-1. Comparison of light sources used in microarray scanners.

Light Sources	Description	Advantages	Disadvantages
Gas Laser	• Gas-filled tube • Fixed wavelength	• Commonly available • Available in specific wavelengths	• Large • Generates heat • Fragile • Inefficient • Uncontrollable
Solid State Laser	• Solid-state semi-conductor crystal • Fixed wavelength	• Small • Efficient • Controllable • Long Life	• Choice of blue wavelengths currently limited
White Light Source	• Xenon arc light source • Range of wavelengths from about 350nm to 750nm or more	• One source for multiple excitations	• Large • Generates a huge quantity of heat • Fragile • Needs filters to block out unwanted wavelengths. • Not as intense as laser source.

3.5 Elimination of Light-Induced Photobleaching

Photobleaching is the permanent chemical destruction of the fluorophore caused by extended exposure to light. This phenomenon occurs when the molecules are excited with a large amount of incident energy. Alternatively, this can occur when the molecules are excited with the large amount of incident energy all at once, or when the molecules are exposed to a modest amount of energy over a long period of time. Fluorophores can only be excited a certain number of times (on average) before they lose the ability to fluoresce. For example, it is widely known that fluorescein can be excited about 30,000 times on average before it is destroyed[1]. Comparison of various excitation strategies is presented in Table 3-2.

Use of excessive laser power is known to cause photobleaching of the dye-labeled features on the microarray substrate. A typical 1 to 20 milli-Watt laser is capable of repeatedly exciting a fluorophore molecule many orders of magnitude beyond the photobleaching level in one second. Therefore, scanners with such features offer an advantage. One example is the *Virtek ChipReader*™, which reaches high levels of sensitivity without resorting to the excessive use of high laser power.

This undesirable photobleaching effect limits the possibility of re-scanning the substrate multiple times. Re-scanning the substrate is recommended, as it is difficult to evaluate the microarray image quality without comparing multiple scans to determine the optimum parameters that generate the best quality image. High quality images are critical for easy and reliable image analysis. To demonstrate the ChipReader's ability to virtually eliminate photobleaching artifacts, a study was performed in which a dilution series slide was scanned 20 times at maximum laser power, and the signal intensities for both *Cy3* and *Cy5* labeled[1] DNA spots were analyzed for each scan. There was no perceivable photobleaching between the scans. For more information on the experimental protocol, please refer to the Virtek Biotech Technical Note on the negligible photobleaching properties of the ChipReader[2].

Excitation light-induced photobleaching is different from environment-induced dye degradation. It has been observed by many microarray users that the signal intensities of dye-labeled DNA arrayed onto microarray substrates will naturally decrease over time. The effect is usually noticeable after about one week has elapsed since the sample has been prepared. Signal degradation occurs over time even when exposure to ambient light and scanner laser power are both minimized, suggesting that time-related degradation is strongly influenced by chemical factors. The effect of time on reducing signal intensities on

---

[1] *Cy3 and Cy5 are trademarks of Amersham Pharmacia Biotech.*

Table 3-2. Comparison of excitation strategies.

Excitation Strategy	Description	Advantages	Disadvantages
Simultaneous excitation	• Multiple light sources excite multiple dyes in the same pixel at the same time	• Increased scanning speed	• Increased crosstalk • Reduced signal to noise ratio
Pixel shifting	• Multiple light sources excite multiple dyes at different pixels at the same time	• Reduced crosstalk • Increased signal to noise ratio	• Channels misalignment requires image registration • Sub-optimal spot analysis
Fiber Optics	• Fiber optic cables direct the light from an external source to the scanning optics	• Flexible use of multiple, large lasers	• Reduced to achieve high resolution • Inefficient optical power delivery
Gated Laser Scanning Mechanism	• The light sources are turned on and off in a predefined sequence • Only one light source is exciting a fluorophore on one pixel at any given time	• Laser lifetime is extended • Crosstalk is virtually eliminated • Photobleaching is greatly reduced	• Reduced scanning speed

hybridized microarray slides could be due to many factors including atmospheric oxygen and storage temperature *(Figure 3-1)*.

Since increased scanning speed has a direct impact on the instrument throughput, simultaneous scanning techniques are preferred over sequential ones. However, the complications of simultaneous scanning need to be addressed. Some of these are crosstalk and/or lack of image registration.

The ChipReader uses a gated method of scanning microarrays that combines the advantages of simultaneous scanning while avoiding its difficulties. For example, the green (532nm) laser scans across a row of pixels on the array surface during the forward pass, and then it is switched off. At that time, the red

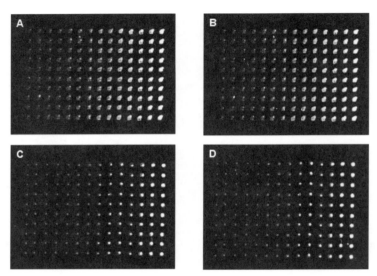

Figure 3-1. A dilution series slide of Cy3-labeled DNA (Figures A and C) and Cy5-labeled DNA (Figures B and D) were scanned 20 consecutive times at maximum laser power to demonstrate the ChipReader does not cause significant photobleaching. The two images on the left-hand side (Figures A and C) are from the first scan, and the two images on the right-habd side (Figures B and D) are from scan number 20.

(635nm) laser starts to scan in the reverse direction across the same row of pixels. Several goals are achieved simultaneously.

- Laser lifetime is extended relative to non-gated lasers.

- Crosstalk caused by simultaneous excitation of two different fluorophores is virtually eliminated.

- Photobleaching is greatly reduced by minimizing the amount of light exposed to the fluorophores.

The latter point on minimizing photobleaching has been taken a further step ahead by using the minimum amount of laser power required to activate the dyes while still achieving the highest sensitivity.

3.6 Optical Design of Confocal Scanners

The impurities normally contained in the coated glass slides used in most microarrays fluoresce in both the Cy3 and Cy5 channels and create a background signal. Also, the excitation light reflected off both the spotted genes and the glass is diffused in all directions inside the scanner. These reflections (stray light) also contribute to the background signal. Furthermore, reflections can occur from below the slide surface as light reflects off of the slide holder and other mechanical parts. Another source of unwanted light is the auto-fluorescence of any and all optical components in the optical path (including the substrate). The fluorescence signal coming from these points is spectrally indistinguishable from the real fluorescence signal from the spots. Therefore, these undesirable sources need to be blocked geometrically with a confocal arrangement. A non-confocal scanner is incapable of discriminating between these unwanted light sources because it collects all of this light, which causes a poorer signal-to-noise ratio when compared to a confocal scanner. Table 3-3 outlines some of the differences between a confocal and non-confocal technology for scanning microarrays. For more information on confocal microscopy and its applications in biology and on the topic of microarray scanners, please consult references [3-7].

The Virtek ChipReader microarray scanner uses confocal optical design to remove stray light and much of the background signal to improve the signal-to-noise ratio and create a better quality image. The depth of focus is pre-set to 25microns to account for unevenness present in the substrate surface (typically on the order of ± 15 microns). Therefore, most confocal microarray scanners

Table 3-3. Comparison between confocal and nonconfocal optical designs.

Optical Design	Description	Advantages	Disadvantages
Confocal	• A pinhole aperture restricts the light collection to the excited area only • Controlled depth of focus	• Blocks out stray light • Greatly reduces background fluorescence signals • Improves signal to noise	• Some focusing require for optimal performance • All-or-none signal when in and out of focus, respectively
Non-confocal	• No pinhole aperture	• No focusing adjustment required • Signal observed irrespective of focus position, albeit corrupt	• Stray excitation light corrupts the signal • Background fluorescence cence contaminates signal • Reduced signal to noise • Artificially high signal intensities due to unwanted addition of non-specific signals

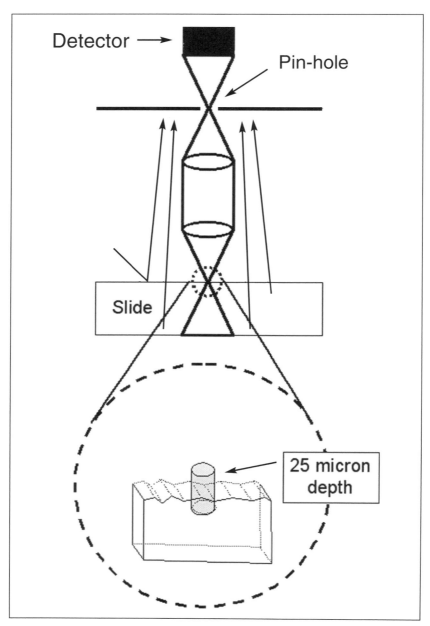

Figure 3-2. Confocal Optical Geometry

are different than a confocal microscope in terms of the depth of focus. A basic schematic of a confocal optical arrangement is presented in *Figure 3-2*.

3.7 Detectors

Two basic types of detectors are used in microarray scanners; photomultiplier tubes (PMT's) and charge-coupled devices (CCD's). These detectors have a light-sensitive component that converts light energy into electronic currents that can be measured. They all have physical limitations concerning the minimum number of photons they can detect. However, the PMT is the most sensitive type of detector available that is small-sized and low-cost relative to a CCD detector that offers similar performance characteristics. Table 3-4 outlines some characteristics of the different detector types.

CCD-based detectors rely on a one-dimensional vector or a two-dimensional array of photosensitive elements. These elements transform incident light into electrical current that can be related to their location in the CCD. Therefore, multiple pixels can be captured at once with a CCD detector. This speeds up the scanning process. However, this is offset by the excessive operational requirements of the CCD's in the context of fluorescence measurements. Namely, in order to achieve the typically required sensitivities, the CCD's need to be cooled to lower the high background noise. despite the large number of pixels that are contained in typical CDCD array, there are not enough present to image the entire microarray surface at high resolution, and therefore several smaller images must be taken and stitched together. As described above, this increases the danger of destroying the sample by photobleaching.

On the other hand, PMT's are designed to detect ultraviolet, visible, and near-infrared light at very low radiant power, and are very sensitive. Incoming photons of the incident excitation light impact a photosensitive electrode surface that emits a proportional quantity of electrons. The emitted electrons then travel inside the tube and strike additional electrodes that generate many more electrons. This process is repeated, perhaps seven to ten times. The end-effect is a huge amplification of the original number of electrons. The PMT's ability to amplify weak signals makes it the most sensitive and suitable optical detection device for microarray scanners. PMT's also have an extremely fast response time.

PMT's generally are manufactured to have a maximum sensitivity for a specific range of wavelengths. Therefore, no single type of PMT is optimally sensitive across the entire spectrum. PMT's have a non-uniform response across their spectral range, and they are more efficient for certain regions of the spectrum, depending on how they are manufactured. Since microarray applications use specific dyes, the fluorescence emission is effectively pre-determined. The fluorescence emissions from these dyes are not scanned as discrete wavelengths to generate a spectral profile as would normally be done in a spectrofluorimeter experiment. Instead, filters are used to collect a spectral range of fluorescence emissions, to be detected as a single emission channel for a particular dye. The goal is to collect as much light as possible over as much of the fluorescence emission spectral curve as possible to increase the detection sensitivity. A different set of filters would be used to detect a second dye. Therefore, the fact that PMT's have a non-uniform response favors the use of specifically selected PMT's to match the dyes in question. However, this discussion illustrates why it is important in microarray applications to choose dyes that do not

Table 3-4. Characteristics of detector types.

Detectors	Description	Advantages	Disadvantages
Single Photo-multiplier tube (PMT)	• Single detection element for one pixel at a time • One PMT for one or more dyes	• The most sensitive type of light detector available • Wide dynamic range • Extremely fast	• The PMTs selective spectral response compromises channel sensitivity • Forces sequential scanning of multiple dyes
Multiple Photo-multiplier tubes (PMT)	• Single detection element for one pixel at a time • Two or more PMTs for more than on channel (simultaneously, or at different times)	• The most sensitive type of light detector available • Wide dynamic range • Extremely fast • Individual and spectrally optimized PMTs for each channel gives maximum sensitivity	• More complex optical design
Charge coupled device (CCD)	• Multiple detection elements for many pixels at a time	• Up to hundreds of thousand of pixels can be accessed at one time	• CCDs are usually 12-bit, and must be "interpolated" to emulate 16-bit • Multiple images must be stitched together to complete a high-resoluiton scan of entire microarray •Require cooling

have a significant degree of spectral overlap. This argument applies for all CCD-based and other microarray scanners as well. Scanners that use a single PMT to cover a wide spectral range of several dyes are, therefore, less adequate, and usually not optimally sensitive. If two different PMT's are used, then each can be selected to have optimal sensitivity for the particular fluorescent dye of interest. This ensures the highest sensitivity and optimal match between the dye emission and the detection system's response.

3.8 Scanning Mechanism

As the name "scanner" implies, either the optics must move across the microarray surface to generate an image, or the slide itself must be moved relative to the stationary optics. The optimal design is the one which uses light-weight moving components when speed is required (Table 3-5). Light-weight lends itself readily to rapid acceleration and deceleration movements, as would be expected in a rapidly moving scanning mechanism. The key issue is positional accuracy. It is much easier to accurately position light-weight moving optics than it is to move a much heavier slide and its holding mechanism quickly and accurately. The ChipReader uses a light-weight moving optical assembly

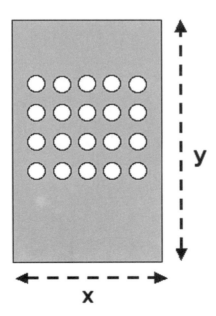

Figure 3-3. Orientation of the slide and labeling of the axis.

Table 3-5. Comparison of scanning mechanisms.

Scanning Mechanism	Description	Advantages	Disadvantages
Slow-moving slide, Fast moving optics	• Slide is stationary in the width direction, and optics is scanned sideways to cover the entire region of interest	• Perfect image registration between channels • Repeatable positioning between scans	• More design effort
Fast moving slide	• Slide is scanned sideways and longitudinally relative to the optics to cover the entire region of interest	• Less design effort	• Uncontrollable repositioning errors between scans • Poor registration

that moves rapidly in a linear direction across the "*x*" dimension of the slide surface *(Figure 3-3)*. It was stated earlier in the section on excitation strategies that the Virtek ChipReader uses a gated scanning mechanism in which only one laser is turned on at any one time during the forward and reverse passes across the row of pixels. After both channels have been collected, the slide holder mechanism advances the slide forward in the "*y*" direction so the next row of data can be collected. Not all scanners work in this manner. Some scanners move the slide in both the "*x*" and "*y*" dimensions relative to stationary optics. It is difficult to quickly move the slide back and forth and simultaneously retain accurate registration.

Laser confocal microarray scanners offer excellent sensitivity, signal-to-noise ratios, and high resolution capabilities. Combined with stable solid-state laser light sources, sensitive - yet affordable - photomultiplier tube detectors, and stable solid holder and scanning mechanisms, the confocal design is very robust and yields high quality images.

References

1. *Singer V, Johnson I*: Fluorophore Characteristics: Making Intelligent Choices in Application-Specific Dye Selection. *Eighth International Symposium on Human Identification* 1997,
http://www.promega.com/geneticidproc/ussymp8proc/21.html

2. This application note is available at **http://www.virtekvision.com**

3. *Pawley JB (ed.):* Handbook of Biological Confocal Microascopy, 2nd edition, *Plenum Press*, NY, 1995.

4. *Paddock SW (ed.):*, Confocal Microscopy Methods and Protocols, Metods in Molecular Biology Series, *Humana Press*, 1998.

5. *Sheppard CJR , Shotton DM :* Confocal laser Scanning Microscopy, Bios Scientific Publishers, *Springer* 1997

6. *Schena M (ed.):* Microarray Biochip technology, BioTechniques Books, *Eaton Publishing,* 2000.

7. *Rampal JB (ed.):* DNA Arrays, Methods and Protocols, Methods in Molecular Biology, vol 170, *Humana Press*, Totowa, NJ, 2000.

CHAPTER 4

CONSIDERATIONS FOR A QUALITY MICROARRAY SCANNER

Scott J. Vacha, Jeffrey McMillan *and* Andreas Dorsel

Contact:
Scott J. Vacha, Ph.D.

Agilent Technologies, 13017 Wisteria Dr. #600, Germantown, Maryland 20874 U.S.A.
E-mail: Scott_Vacha@agilent.com

0-9664027-5-8/02/$0.00+$.50   *From:* **Microarray Image Analysis-Nuts & Bolts** (pp.69-82)
©2002 by DNA Press, LLC   Edited by: S. Shah and G. Kamberova

4.1 Introduction

In all biological experiments data quality is a function of both experimental design and the research tools used in the experimental process. For microarray experiments, these tools involve target labeling, microarray manufacturing, microarray hybridization, scanning, image-analysis, and higher-level bioinformatics. Given this multi-step process, it is crucial for meaningful biological interpretations that the resulting data are a reflection of differential gene expression and not the variability of system components. Although individual tools may incrementally contribute to the overall process, an optimized 'solutions approach' is recommended for microarray experiments. This chapter highlights the technical aspects of one component, the microarray scanner, for new users adopting microarray technology. Although intended as a general introduction, several features of Agilent's SureScan Technology will be introduced.

4.2 Scanner Overview

As array technology transitioned to glass substrate from nylon-based arrays (for advantages in throughput, scale, image acquisition, and two-color hybridization see[1]), new instrumentation became necessary to measure the fluorophores used in target labeling (typically Cyanine-3 and Cyanine-5). To that end, all scanners were designed to measure the amount of fluorescence emitted from a microarray slide. However, because an underlying assumption is made that the quantity of fluorophores in a given location (feature, or DNA spot) correlates to the level of endogenous gene transcription, it is important to obtain an accurate measurement of this fluorescent signal. Consequently, scanner specifications (regarding sensitivity, uniformity, resolution, throughput, dynamic range and cross-talk) are important for selecting a quality optical instrument. In addition, engineering improvements to reduce noise and image-extraction algorithms to estimate noise have important implications for detecting subtle differences in gene expression with confidence based on statistical analysis.

In general, microarray scanners fall into two main categories, those that use charged-coupled devices (CCD's) and others that use laser light with photomultiplier tube (PMT) detection. CCD's commonly use flood-illumination (e.g. a broadband Xenon arc lamp) to simultaneously acquire a microarray image that is divided into pixels by the detector. Because a CCD detector cannot acquire the entire dimension of a microarray slide with high resolution, smaller regions are typically scanned and 'stitched' together by software to improve image quality [2]. The longer exposure time necessary to improve resolution and subsequent software manipulation may have implications on array photobleaching and image integrity. In addition, the use of flood illumination typically results in a higher background illumination from the glass substrate and the opposite slide surface, as it prevents rejection of these undesired sources of background (e.g. by depth discrimination). Point-source illumination (a laser spot of essentially constant power scanned across the sample) typically results in better spatial uniformity of the measurement. Although a CCD-based system may compensate for signal magnitude variations by post-processing the data, it cannot compensate for the resulting variation in shot-noise.

The more commonly used scanner technology involves laser excitation and PMT detection to build microarray images pixel by pixel via raster scanning. Here, well-defined wavelengths of laser light, corresponding to the excitation peaks of incorporated fluorophores, are directed to the microarray slide in a simultaneous or sequential fashion. As the fluorophore-labeled target is excited, the emitted photons impinge upon a photocathode material (PC) to cause photoelectron (PE) emission. The PE charge is then amplified by multiple dynodes to produce a current pulse that is proportional to the amount of incident light[3]. The fraction of impinging photons that result in photoelectrons and contribute to the output signal is referred to as the quantum efficiency Q_E of the PMT (not to be confused with the quantum efficiency of the dye). Often, confocal or other depth-discriminating optical designs are combined with PMT detection to ensure that only photons emitted from a defined plane of focus (i.e. the microarray features) are quantified. This increases scanner sensitivity by eliminating out-of-focus light not originating from the targets of interest. For state-of-the-art systems, this results in a lower limit of detection, equivalent to higher sensitivity. Given the typically increased sensitivity and resolution of laser scanning and PMT detection compared to CCD-based systems, this chapter will focus on PMT-based scanner technology.

4.3 Instrumental Noise

One of the challenges in microarray-based experiments is to minimize and account for noise in the overall process such that subtle differences can be attributed to biological changes and not to instrumental or process variability. Although all microarray scanners will generate an image, instrumentation that offers minimal noise, good uniformity, high sensitivity and error modeling can help minimize the downstream effort and resources spent pursuing false leads. Given the dollar value of each microarray data point (RNA kits, labeling kits, microarrays, labor, bioinformatics) and the cost of downstream applications based upon these data (TaqMan®, RT-PCR, cellular assays, labor), a quality data measurement tool can be a wise investment. This section highlights some of the sources of noise in scanner technology, independent of chemical or biological noise.

4.3.1 Shot Noise

In microarray scanners, where individual photons of light are detected, intrinsic limitations exist due to the particle nature of light. Here, the Poisson statistics of molecules hybridized per pixel and of photons detected per molecule limit the accuracy of measuring these quantum-mechanical events[3]. As signal intensity increases, so does the level of shot noise, albeit proportional to the square root of the signal[2]. Although this type of noise cannot be eliminated from any scanner, it can be estimated and accounted for in the data extraction error model. In well-designed optical systems, all other sources of instrumental noise are minimized such that shot noise is the major contributor[4]. It should be noted, that the square-root dependence of noise on signal described above has its limitations: If signal is increased by integrating over more detected photons, the overall signal-to-noise ratio changes from being limited by photon statistics to being limited by molecular statistics[5]. For example, if only one photon is detected on average per hybridized molecule, then the resulting signal-to-noise is already close to 70% of the limit set by the number of molecules present.

4.3.2 PMT Noise

As described earlier, PMT's detect fluorophore-emitted photons and amplify the signal through a series of dynodes to produce a current pulse. Fluctuations in this signal amplification that are not reflective of the initial photon emission are considered PMT excess noise. This is a multiplicative noise. Dark current of a PMT (or other detector) may cause additional noise. Dark current may result from leakage currents between the electrodes, thermal PE emission from the dynodes, or thermally excited PE's leaving the PC[3]. This dark current noise and electronic noise is sometimes referred to as the *additive noise* in the detector[4]. Furthermore, poor signal amplification and digitizing circuitry can contribute additional noise in poorly designed systems. High quality components, precision engineering and low noise design can minimize the contribution of PMT and electronic noise to the overall measurement.

Because PMT gain/sensitivity is partially dependent upon an applied voltage, many commercial microarray scanners enable users to adjust this voltage with each slide. This allows users to increase the intensity of dim features on a microarray, or to decrease the intensity of saturated features. Although researchers may prefer visibly bright arrays, it should be noted that both signal and background intensity increase proportionally with increased PMT voltage. This means that researchers will typically not improve the signal-to-noise ratio of an array by increasing the PMT voltage, unless system noise was dominated by additive electronic noise or digitization noise which typically occurs for poorly designed systems only[2]. At *very* low PMT gain, the PMT excess noise may become noticeable too. In addition, adjusting PMT voltages often becomes a process of trial and error, as there is a highly non-linear relationship between PMT voltage and the resulting signal levels that a user sees in the image file. Even different PMT's from the same manufacturing lot can produce widely different results with the same applied voltage. For this reason, Agilent's SureScan technology is unique in offering linear PMT control whereby researchers can adjust the PMT sensitivity level. When a different scale factor is selected by the user, the scanner automatically adjusts the PMT voltages accordingly (Figure 4-1). This eliminates the need for multiple re-scans.

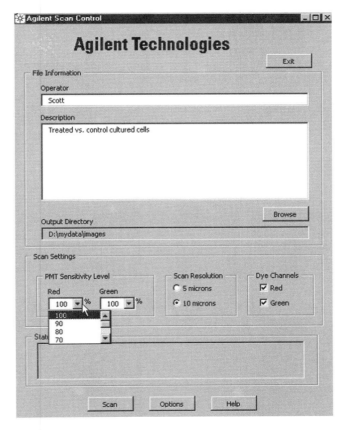

Figure 4-1. **User PMT control:** Agilent's SureScan technology offers intuitive PMT control that ensures a linear relationship between PMT voltage and the resulting image density. This figure illustrates the user-defined PMT settings in a pull down menu.

4.3.3 Laser Noise

In quantifying the fluorescent emission of microarray features, an assumption is made that the level of fluorescence is proportional to the amount of endogenous gene transcription. Because the level of fluorescence is also proportional the amount of laser light falling on the array, it is important to compensate for laser drift over time. Noise in the laser can contribute to noise in the image, all other things being equal. Without laser monitoring and control, users may detect decreased microarray intensity over the life of the laser or even intensity fluctuations over the course of a single scan. Although some lasers can self-correct for temperature fluctuations or compensate for long-term laser light drift, these *internal* sensors respond in minutes and cannot compensate for real-time fluctuations. To maintain data integrity over the course of a single scan and consistent intensities over the life of the laser, users should consider scanners with *external* laser power modulation as well (Figure 4-2). This ensures that a uniform intensity of laser light will be applied to all features on the same microarray. In addition, external laser modulation virtually eliminates the long-term signal drift due to laser aging and enables calibration across scanners. This is critical for high throughput facilities where obtaining comparable results across multiple microarray scans and scanners is important.

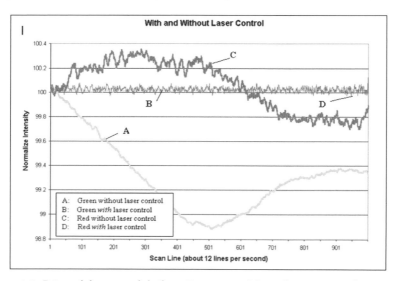

Figure 4-2. **External laser modulation:** Two sequential 7 minute scans of a standard 1"x3" glass slide. The data illustrates up to a 20-fold improvement in laser stability for the Agilent SureScan system over the uncompensated data, resulting in more uniform laser intensity across the microarray slide.

4.3.4 Non-Uniformity

While scanning microarray slides in the X and Y-direction, microarray scanners must also track the slides' surface in the Z-direction. This maximizes scanner sensitivity by restricting measurements to the light emitted from DNA features on or close to the microarray surface, rather than out-of-focus light. In the absence of autofocus, spatial non-uniformity of sensitivity across the scan image can occur. This may result in artifacts that add to signal noise or, worse still, cause a bias that may be mistaken for a biological change. This source of noise is important to consider because the glass surface of microarrays varies in thickness, surface roughness, and curvature. It has been reported that typical glass slides can have 18 microns or greater in surface variability (Z-direction) leading to 25-30% variability in signal intensity[6]. If the scanner cannot accurately measure DNA features in the focal plane, then sensitivity, uniformity, and data integrity will be compromised.

Some scanner manufacturers address this issue by widening the field of focus (depth discrimination). Although this approach addresses the surface variability, it decreases the overall scanner sensitivity by measuring light that does not originate from the DNA features of interest. Other manufacturers optimize the slide positioning in order to narrow the depth discrimination. Although this ensures maximal sensitivity for features within the set plane of focus, it does not account for curvature or variability in the glass surface. As a result, signal intensity will decrease for out-of-focus features (Figure 4-3). This reflects poorly on the scanner's field uniformity and data integrity because the X-Y position of DNA features now becomes important in the resulting signal intensity.

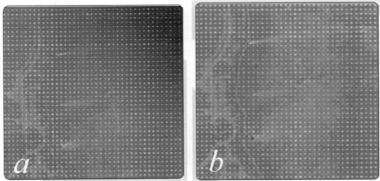

Figure 4-3. **The importance of focus.** This figure shows a portion of a microarray image toggled to log scale in order to visualize the slide surface. Figure *a* illustrates the array scanned at a defined focal plane to show the effect of surface curvature/variability on the resulting signal intensity (note features in upper right image). Figure *b* shows the same microarray with Agilent's Dynamic Autofocus, which ensures that every feature on the microarray is in focus.

Poor scanner uniformity can be detected by scanning a microarray slide in one direction, turning the slide 180 degrees for re-scanning in the other direction, and comparing the data (Figure 4-4). Because variability in log ratios resulting from instrumentation can compromise the statistical confidence with which scientists measure differential gene expression, field uniformity specifications are important in selecting a quality microarray scanner.

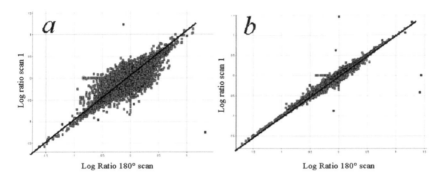

Figure 4-4. **The effects of scanner non-uniformity**. This figure shows data-extracted log ratios of a microarray scanned in one orientation compared to the same array rotated 180° and re-scanned. *(a)* Results obtained from a competing scanner indicate non-uniformity, with an R^2 value of 0.697 and a slope of $Y=0.819*X-0.00237$ *(b)* The same experiment on Agilent's scanner resulted in an R^2 value of 0.984 and slope of $Y=0.989*X-0.000705$. The features labeled in blue were flagged by the software for hybridization non-uniformity. By eliminating the positional variability due to surface non-uniformity, users can have confidence that detected differences are a function of biology and not instrumentation. (Data points grouped in conspicuous lines along the x and y axis are caused by the analysis software setting the log ratio to 0 for negative numbers obtained when surrounding background is higher than the signal from a feature.)

Agilent's SureScan technology introduces the first Dynamic Autofocus in microarray scanning. This means that the scanner can detect and compensate for subtle variations in the microarray surface, making micron-level adjustments (Z-direction) in sub-millisecond response (Figure 4-5). By maintaining tight depth discrimination and making up to 1 million dynamic adjustments over the course of a single scan, Agilent's microarray scanner can ensure that every feature is within focus with maximum sensitivity. This enables a global non-uniformity specification of 5% RMS with a lower limit of detection than competing scanners. It also improves the statistical confidence of microarray results by eliminating focal plane noise as a source of variability.

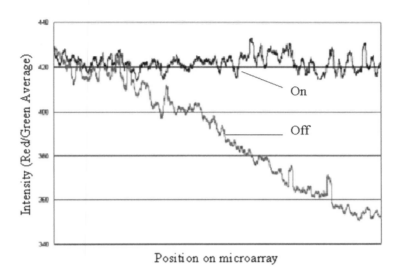

Figure 4-5. **Agilent's dynamic autofocus.** A comparison of horizontal cuts between rows of features near the top of the image on each microarray scan from Figures 3a,b shows a decrease in the background (resulting from incomplete washing or glass curvature) in the scan with the dynamic autofocus feature disabled (OFF). The same microarray scanned with the dynamic autofocus feature enabled shows no decrease (ON).

4.4 Sensitivity and Resolution

Increased sensitivity is considered a beneficial characteristic in the microarray process, as DNA microarrays are typically used for discovery purposes (pattern discovery, functional discovery, target discovery). Although genes showing high differential expression will likely be detected on most platforms, scientists are typically interested in capturing as much information as possible under a set experimental condition. It has been shown that microarray targets can exhibit statistically significant changes in gene expression below a 1.5-fold threshold. Even at low target abundance these changes can have biological relevance that contributes to experimental interpretation and correlation[7]. Although sensitivity is partially a function of the microarray platform, the microarray scanner can make a positive contribution toward detecting low-abundant transcripts with high confidence.

In the context of DNA microarrays, sensitivity refers to the minimum number of fluorophores per unit area that a scanner can detect for a given pixel, equivalent to the ability of the scanner to detect signal over background noise. By coating a microarray slide with fluorophores in a well-defined experimental procedure, precision calculations can be obtained for the lower limit of scanner detection. Microarray scanner manufacturers typically report this number as chromophores per square micron (cpsm), or the minimum number of dye molecules per 10 micron pixel (Figure 4-6). A smaller cpsm specification corresponds to a more sensitive instrument.

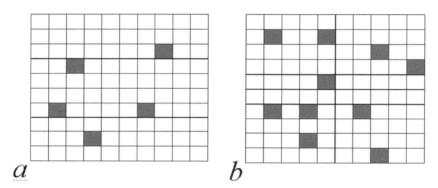

Figure 4-6. **CPSM measurements.** This figure represents the minimum number of dye molecules (black boxes) that can be detected by a scanner at a 10-micron pixel resolution. Panel *a* represents the detection limit of a scanner at 0.05 cpsm compared to the detection limit of a less sensitive instrument (0.1 cpsm, *b*). The ability to detect a smaller number of dye molecules in a given region (Figure 4-6a) means that scientists can obtain meaningful data from low-abundance transcripts.

As stated, sensitivity corresponds to a scanner's ability to detect signal over background noise. If there is a large standard deviation in background noise, the software will be less able to distinguish DNA fluorescence from the noise of the background[2]. One way to measure this is to plot the distribution of pixels in a uniform background region, such as a blank slide (Figure 4-7). Uniform regions should result in uniform data. In this context it is important to have a sufficient offset (not be confused with background) on the signal, so that unclipped raw data are available as a prerequisite to meaningful analysis.

In addition to signal-to-noise or detection limit and spatial uniformity of scans, reproducibility over time (or temporal uniformity) is also necessary in order to obtain reliable data. Here, improved uniformity enables multiple scanners to be calibrated for use in a high throughput environment. This can be measured by scanning a single array multiple times and comparing the data consistency across scans.

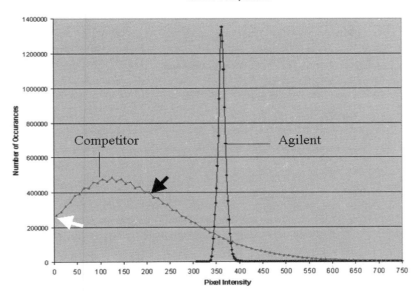

Figure 4-7. **Background noise.** This figure illustrates the distribution of pixels on a blank slide scanned on the Agilent scanner and a competing scanner with appropriate scaling. The high background noise of the competing scanner, as indicated by the broad distribution of background pixels, will impact sensitivity and limit the scanner's ability to discern signal over background. The saw-tooth pattern of the curve (black arrow) indicates problems with pre-amplification/digitization circuitry or faulty data processing. Finally, this competing scanner throws out data by clipping data points at low intensity (white arrow) while the Agilent data indicates an offset intended to avoid clipping of data in the presence of noise. Clipping data can result in loss of data on dim features.

The term sensitivity is often confused with pixel 'resolution', which refers to the fineness of detail or distance between data points collected by the scanner. Many commercial scanners offer 5-10 micron resolution to acquire sufficient data from microarray features. Higher resolution scans provide more data points for statistics (unless the laser diameter is larger than the pixel size which creates an inaccurate pixel map), but result in significantly larger data files. For this reason users typically compromise, while keeping the resolution lower than 1/8-1/10 the feature diameter (e.g. 10-micron resolution for a 100-micron feature).

4.5 Throughput

Most microarray experiments involve the use of tens to hundreds of arrays to profile experimental conditions, time courses, or drug targets. For this reason, a good microarray scanner should also incorporate features that improve the throughput of microarray scanning and data analysis. The amount of time that researchers dedicate to single-load scanners or non-automated image analysis tools is time that could be better spent on biological research and experimentation. Because it can take up to two hours for experienced users to completely process a single array on some systems (scan time, spot finding, grid overlay, feature flagging, data analysis), improvements in throughput can have a positive impact on the labor costs involved in running a microarray facility.

From an instrument standpoint, throughput can be improved by selecting a scanner with multi- loading capability. This can be a slide holder or carousel that automates the loading and scanning of microarray slides. Even if users do not completely fill the carousel it offers a significant time benefit, compared to returning to the scanner every few minutes for slide handling.

From a software standpoint, throughput can be improved by automating the image analysis. This includes automating image overlay, feature finding, grid overlay, feature flagging, background subtraction, normalization, error modeling, log ratio calculations, and data output. The underlying algorithms should be based on sound statistics that combine systematic error estimation, objective feature flagging and non-uniformity measurements with user-defined statistical thresholds to output log ratios, P-values and error bars in a user-friendly format. Data obtained using defined statistical cutoffs with P-values and error bars avoids combining experiments that have been subjectively flagged and analyzed by multiple researchers over time.

Agilent's microarray scanner and feature extraction software address both bottlenecks by offering automated scanning (up to 48 slides per carousel) and automated data extraction. When using Agilent microarrays, the extraction software can automatically perform feature finding, feature/background flagging (for saturation, non-uniformity, population outlier), background subtraction, dye normalization, and log ratio calculations with P-values and error bars for a single array, all in less than 1 minute[8]. Combined with the throughput capabilities of the carousel and the internal barcode reader/data management tools, this drastically reduces the time from experiment to analysis and enables researchers to focus on biology[9].

4.6 Summary

Because all microarray scanners can generate an image, users are not always cognizant of the contribution that a quality instrument can make to the overall microarray process. Projects that involve 'gene-fishing' for extreme outliers will likely succeed on any instrument, as subtle differences in instrument noise will not likely mask this 'low-hanging fruit'. However, as scientists recognize the long-term need for expression analysis in their research, as more powerful bioinformatics tools succeed in simplifying the complexity of gene expression patterns, and as pharmaceutical companies establish guidelines for consistent microarray processes, the benefits of high quality instrumentation will become more apparent.

A quality scanner should produce consistent results with high sensitivity and uniformity, while minimizing the contribution of instrument variability to the overall microarray process. Issues such as field uniformity, cross-talk, sensitivity, laser control, dynamic autofocus, and throughput should all be considered. As with any scientific experiment, the resulting data is a function of experimental design and the tools used to generate it. By minimizing systematic variability, researchers will have confidence that the observed changes are a function of biology and not components of the microarray process.

References

1. *Southern E, Mir K, Shchepinov M*: Molecular interactions on microarrays. *Nature Genet. Suppl.* 1999; 21: 5-9.

2. *Basarsky T, Verdnik D, Zhai J Ye, Wellis D*: Overview of a microarray scanner: Design essentials for an integrated acquisition and analysis platform. in Schena M (ed): *Microarray Biochip Technology*, Eaton, Natick, 2000, pp. 265-284.

3. *Pawley JB*: Sources of noise in three-dimensional microscopical data sets: in Stevens JK, Mills LR, Trogadis JE (eds): Three-Dimensional Confocal Microscopy: Volume Investigation of Biological Systems, San Diego, *Academic Press*, 1996, pp. 47-69.

4. *Pawley JB*: Fundamental limits in confocal microscopy. in Pawley JB (ed): title. Handbook of Biological Confocal Microscopy, 2nd Ed, New York, *Plenum Press*, 1995, pp.19-37.

5. *Dorsel A*: Fundamental Performance Limitations of Hybridized Arrays, Invited Paper, Lake Tahoe Symposion on *Microarray Algorithms and Statistical Analysis: Methods and Standards* 1999.

6. *Handran S, Wang C, Aziz D*: Assessing Slide Flatness. Application note available at: **http://www.axon.com/genomics/Assessing_Slide_Flatness.pdf**

7. *Hughes TR et al.*: Functional Discovery via a compendium of expression profiles. *Cell* 2000; 102: 109-126.

8. *Delenstarr G et al*: Estimating the confidence limits of oligonucleotide microarray-based measurements of differential expression. Pub.# 5988-2362EN, 2001; Available through **http://www.agilent.com/chem/dna**,

9. Visit **http://www.agilent.com** to learn more about Agilent's developments in microarray technology

KEY CONSIDERATIONS FOR ACCURATE MICROARRAY SCANNING AND IMAGE ANALYSIS

Damian Verdnik, Shawn Handran *and* Siobhan Pickett
Axon Instruments, Inc.

Contact:

Axon Instruments, Inc., 3280 Whipple Road, Union City, CA 94587 U.S.A.
Phone: (510) 675-6200 Fax: (510) 675-6300
www.axon.com

0-9664027-5-8/02/$0.00+$.50   *From:* **Microarray Image Analysis-Nuts & Bolts** (pp.83-98)
©2002 by DNA Press, LLC   Edited by: S. Shah and G. Kamberova

5.1 Introduction

Microarrays are rapidly becoming a standard experimental tool in biomedical research. Expression profiling, a technique pioneered by Brown and colleagues[1], employs quantitative fluorescence imaging and analysis to compare the hybridization of two differentially labeled mRNA expression libraries to DNA probes of interest that have been spotted in an array, typically on standard glass microscope slides. The power of microarray technology lies in the ability to analyze and compare many thousands of individual samples simultaneously. The technology has been applied to nucleic acids, proteins, whole cells, tissue sections, and different types of small molecules. The parallel analysis of thousands of samples across many arrays can provide a more comprehensive understanding of the complex interactions that drive biological processes than any other experimental method available to date. It is no wonder that more and more investigators in a wide range of disciplines are adopting the technique. This chapter reviews how to obtain the most reliable performance from the microarray scanner, and discusses several image analysis methods used in microarray experiments, including numerical pre-processing methods that can be considered prior to cluster analysis of large sets of microarray data.

5.2 Calibration

Any scientific instrument must perform consistently over time so that results can be compared from day to day and week to week. In addition, in a laboratory that uses several identical instruments, given the same sample each instrument must give the same results. However mechanical and electronic components have a finite lifetime, so performance will change as the instrument ages. A calibrated instrument ensures experimental reproducibility both over time and among different instruments. The consequence for microarray scanner design is that the instrument must be able to be calibrated.

Calibrating an instrument can involve a number of different procedures, but fundamentally it involves matching the performance of the instrument to a known standard. For fluorescence imaging, this entails adjusting the instrument to produce a specified signal output from the known fluorescent standard. The notion of "standard fluorescence" can mean one of two things:

- Standard fluorescence from a ratio channel;

- Standard fluorescence from a monochromatic channel.

Depending on what one means by standard fluorescence, one needs to perform two different calibration procedures.

5.2.1 Calibrating a Ratio Channel

A ratio channel is a data channel that is obtained by dividing two raw acquisition channels. In the standard two-color, red-green ratiometric microarray experiment that we are discussing here, the ratio channel is the channel obtained by dividing the red image by the green image.

Calibrating the ratio channel means adjusting the sensitivity of the detectors in the instrument so that when we measure a red-green ratio of 1.0, it corresponds to a ratio of 1.0 between the red and green fluorescent dyes in the sample. For many microarrays this is a simple procedure, as across the whole slide, most genes are not differentially expressed, and as many genes are over-expressed as under-expressed. This means that the average ratio of intensity across the whole slide should be approximately 1.

In a laser scanning system that uses photomultiplier tubes (PMT's) to amplify the fluorescent signal, ratio calibration adjusts the gain applied to the PMT's. In GenePix Pro™, the software that controls Axon Instruments' GenePix™ series scanners, it is a simple procedure to adjust PMT voltage and observe the change to the total intensity ratio for the slide.

Calibrating the ratio channel only has a number of disadvantages compared with calibrating the individual fluorescent channels:

• Not all experiments are ratiometrics;

• Not all samples lean themselves to it. Experiments on subsets of genes selected for over-expression or under-expression may produce arrays that are heavily skewed to one color. If one does not know the actual ratio of intensities across the whole slide, one must use a set of calibration spots or a separate calibration slide for each ratio channel.

• To perform stringent quality control on large batches of microarrays, the absolute amount of fluorescence in a single channel is an important quality control criterion.

• Balancing the detectors for each channel does not mean that one is acquiring the optimal amount of signal in each channel. That is, one may not be using the entire dynamic range of the instrument (see below, 'Maximizing Dynamic Range').

For all these reasons, the ability to calibrate individual fluorescent channels is an essential of microarray scanner design and use.

5.2.2 Calibrating Individual Channels

GenePix scanners employ a proprietary calibration procedure using calibration slides to calibrate each wavelength channel independently. These calibration slides are optimized for fluorescence with different laser excitation wavelengths, and exhibit negligible photobleaching. GenePix scanners are calibrated in the factory so that each scanner gives the same response in each channel to the same amount of incident fluorescence, and with the click of a button users can periodically calibrate their scanners for repeatable PMT performance over long periods of time.

5.3 Detection Limit

One of the most common misconceptions about microarray imaging is that a brighter image is a better image. However, the absolute brightness of an image tells us nothing about how well features can be distinguished from background. An apparently faint image in which features are clearly differentiated from background is more useful than a bright image in which the features are indistinguishable from the background.

Microarray scanners are fluorescence detection systems: they illuminate a microarray slide, gather emitted fluorescence, amplify and digitize the signal and record the image as a high-resolution image file. Fluorescence imaging and digital signal processing are not new technologies, so while microarray scanners might be relatively new, the mathematical, physics and engineering principles on which they are based have been used in commercial scientific instruments for decades. In particular, the criterion for measuring the detection limit of a fluorescent imaging system is well established. This criterion is *signal-to-noise ratio*, which is the ability of the instrument to detect signal (in this case, fluorescent dye bound to the arrayed biomolecules) above background (the microarray slide). By using signal-to-noise ratio as the final arbiter of microarray data quality, we have a method of judging the absolute performance of a microarray scanning system.

The signal-to-noise ratio (SNR) quantifies how well one can resolve a true signal from the noise of the system. It is typically expressed as the background-corrected peak signal divided by the variation in the background ('noise'):

SNR = (Signal - Background) / (Standard Deviation of Background)

This quantity is commonly used in many signal-processing disciplines, including radio, electronics, and imaging. It tells us that SNR can be increased by increasing the signal measurement, decreasing the background, or decreasing the background standard deviation.

A commonly accepted criterion for the minimum signal that can be accurately quantified (i.e. the detection limit) is the sample value for which the signal is three times greater than the background noise:

$$SNR = 3 = Detection\ Limit$$

Below this point features may be visible, but the ability to accurately quantify them diminishes.

The signal-to-noise ratio of your microarray data is ultimately determined by the cumulative contribution of each step of the arraying process, including array creation, fluorescent excitation, signal collection, image generation, data extraction, and results analysis. Many of these contributions occur inside your microarray scanner, such as the methods of light delivery to the sample, light collection from the sample, optical design, optical detectors, amplifiers and digitizers (for a discussion see [2], [3]). Therefore, to maximize the signal-to-noise ratio of your microarray images, one of the most important decisions you can make is in your choice of microarray scanner. When buying a scanner it is wise to have the same microarray slide scanned on a number of competing scanners to determine the scanner that produces the best signal-to-noise ratio. Axon Instruments' GenePix Pro software includes a number of tools to analyze microarray images and report the overall signal-to-noise ratio, making such scanner-to-scanner comparisons easy.

Once you have made your choice of scanner, there are still some important aspects of the microarraying process under your control. Taking steps to maximize SNR improves the accuracy of the data, and ultimately the confidence in interpretation of the results.

5.4 Signal-to-Noise Ratio and Array Creation

Microarray creation is a multi-step process involving surface coating, array target preparation, fluorescent probe preparation, hybridization and stringency washing. One of the most common sources of background signal is the hybridized microarray sample itself. The utmost care must be taken to minimize all sources of background when creating fluorescent microarrays. In addition, the highest possible hybridization signal levels are ensured by proper care of all fluorescent reagents, and by optimizing DNA binding and hybridization conditions. Each of these steps can be optimized to maximize SNR.

Glass microscope slides are commonly used as a convenient support matrix for microarrays created by mechanical deposition. Other types of arrays are also available, and most of the issues discussed here apply to all fluorescent microarrays. There are commercially available microscope slides that are pre-treated for a variety of applications, including microarrays. For microarrays, the glass slides must be coated with a DNA binding agent prior to DNA deposition. Only the highest quality glass and coating reagents should be used. Impurities in low-grade glass and reagents can fluoresce and increase both overall background signal and irregular noise. The coating process must also be carefully controlled to ensure an even reactive surface across the entire working area of the slide. Non-uniform coating can cause irregular target binding, leading to low signal, and/or target loss. Non-uniform coating will also allow variable non-specific DNA binding, thereby causing high and/or irregular background signal.

Most forms of DNA can be bound to appropriately coated glass slides. PCR products and oligonucleotides are the most commonly used samples in mechanical deposition arrayers. Regardless of the DNA type, all samples must be carefully purified prior to arraying. Certain components in common biochemical buffers can inhibit arrayed DNA from binding to the glass. If the inhibition is such that the DNA in the arrayed spots is not in excess relative to the hybridized probe, the signal in the resulting hybridized spot may be low. If the fluorescent hybridizing probe is in excess, signal levels will not accurately represent the expression levels of the hybridized genes. In addition, the DNA binding capacity of glass is lower than that of commonly used blotting membranes, so there may be significant excess arrayed DNA at each spot. Arrayed DNA that is not eliminated prior to hybridization can bind non-specifically to the glass causing increased background. It can also bind to the fluorescent probe in solution, thereby reducing the probe available for specific hybridization, and subsequently reducing the signal level from corresponding genes. Fluorescently labeled hybridizing samples must also be carefully purified after labeling. Unincorporated fluorescent nucleotides and short extension products can increase both background noise and overall background signal. Non-specific hybridization can be minimized by optimizing the hybridization and stringency wash solutions and temperatures. DNA arrayed onto glass does not bind as robustly as DNA on membranes, so conditions must also be designed to avoid washing the arrayed samples off the slides.

Fluorescent compounds absorb and emit light of different wavelengths with different efficiencies. As indicated by their characteristic absorption and emission spectra, they absorb energy from a range of wavelengths. Excessive exposure to any light within the absorption spectrum, including white light, can cause photobleaching. All fluorescent components in a microarray experiment must be protected from light whenever practical during each phase of the experiment. As with many biochemicals, repeated freeze-thaw cycles and unfavorable chemical conditions can also degrade fluorescently labeled nucleotides. To maximize signal by promoting efficient probe labeling and hybridization, protect fluorescent compounds from light and follow the manufacturers' handling instructions exactly.

5.4.1 Signal-to-noise ratio and PMT gain

As mentioned above, one of the most common misconceptions about microarray imaging is that a brighter image is a better image. The easiest way to get a brighter image is simply to increase the gain of the PMT's in the scanner. However, as mentioned earlier the most important factor when evaluating image quality is the SNR.

Increasing the gain of the PMT does not necessarily increase the SNR (Figure 5-1). As the PMT gain is increased there is an equivalent increase in the noise. The end result is that there is virtually no change in the SNR. While there can be some argument made that the PMT voltage has to be higher than a minimal value to detect anything at all, there is little point to pushing the PMT voltage to its extremes to get a brighter image.

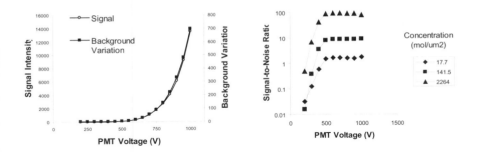

Figure 5-1. Increasing the PMT voltage does not improve the SNR. The panel on the left shows that as the PMT voltage is increased, both the signal and the noise are scaled uniformly. The SNR does not improve as the PMT voltage is increased (right panel).

5.4.2 Signal-to-Noise Ratio and Line Averaging

In contrast to increasing the PMT gain, averaging (or integrating) an image can increase the SNR. For the purposes of this discussion, line averaging is effectively the same as line integration (Figure 5-2). When you repetitively scan the same line, the total amount of signal collected increases linearly as the number of lines to average increases (if you are in line averaging mode, you simply divide this signal by the number of lines averaged). In contrast to the signal, the noise of the system only increases as the square root of the number of lines to average. As a result, as the number of lines averaged or integrated increases, the signal increases in greater proportion than the noise. The end result is a favorable increase in the SNR.

There are two minor disadvantages when using line averaging. The first is that photobleaching increases as more lines are scanned, thus there is a point of diminishing returns, particularly for dim samples or when using fluorophores that are more sensitive to light damage. The second disadvantage is practical: using line averaging increases the scan time. This can become disadvantageous when imaging a large scan area or if faster throughput is desired. Nevertheless, neither of these disadvantages need prevent the use of line averaging, but should be considered and balanced accordingly by the investigator.

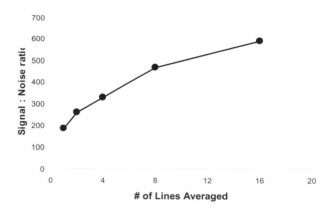

Figure 5-2. Line averaging increases SNR.

5.5 Maximizing Dynamic Range

Dynamic range refers to the number of gradations in a digital detection system that an analog signal can be converted into. For image-forming devices, like the PMT sensor employed in Axon's GenePix scanner, the dynamic range is 16-bit, which is 2^{16}, or 65536 levels. The larger the dynamic range of the detector, the higher the sensitivity since weaker signals (such as those arising from low-copy number transcripts in the case of an expression profile experiment) can be detected without saturating regions of high intensity. That is, a wider dynamic range allows a wider range of dim and bright signals to coexist in the same image with less saturation of the bright features.

In a 16-bit image, each pixel is assigned a value between 0 and 65535, with zero representing no signal and 65535 indicating that the detector has been saturated. Note that there is always some non-zero value (i.e. no pixels will ever have a value of zero) due to the dark current noise of the detection sensor. On the other end of the scale, setting the PMT voltage too high will result in many saturated pixels in the image, indicating that the gain has been set too high for the specimen in question. For best results, the laser power and PMT settings should adjusted so that intensity levels recorded in the image comprise the full dynamic range of the detector. This can be done by adjusting the PMT voltage until a number of pixels are saturated and then slightly decreasing the setting until no pixels in the image are saturated. However, in light of the previous section, one must also balance using a higher PMT voltage with achieving a satisfactory SNR. Under optimal experimental conditions as previously mentioned (e.g. substrate properties, fluorophore labeling, hybridization, wash conditions, etc.), there should be no problem in finding an optimal PMT setting for best SNR while also employing most or all of the dynamic range of the detector. If you are unable to use the full dynamic range because the brightest features do not saturate until the background values become prohibitively high, this sometimes can be an indication of a systematic error or problem in the sample preparation or hybridization process.

5.6 What You Need to Know about Your Scanned Images

The fundamental task to be performed by any first-pass microarray analysis software is the extraction of data from the image produced by the scanner. From the time the microarray slide is placed in the scanner, the user wants the answer to the biological question: is gene *x* over-expressing or under-expressing? What confidence do I have in the result? The analysis software should provide the answers to these questions as seamlessly as possible.

Ideally, the same software that controls the scanner should acquire and analyze the images. Not only does this produce a streamlined workspace, it allows direct and immediate access to the data. With the GenePix scanners, the user can begin to analyze images as they are acquired. In addition, the GenePix workflow options allow the user to concatenate common tasks to proceed automatically.

5.6.1 Scanning Parameters and Quantitation

5.6.1.1 Scan Resolution and Spot Size

Scanner manufacturers routinely advertise the maximum resolution of their scanners, and rightly so, as many microarray users are pushing the limits of scanners by printing smaller and smaller spots. However, for the large majority of microarray users, the maximum resolution of their scanner is more resolution than they need. To reduce image sizes and hence storage and computational requirements, you should always use a resolution that is appropriate for your median spot size. For example, scanning at 5 μm is useful primarily for analysis of features smaller than about 100 μm in diameter. A 100 μm feature scanned with 10 μm pixels contains about 78 pixels, which is sufficient for an accurate intensity measurement. For features larger than 100 μm, the negligible difference in accuracy is unlikely to justify the four-fold increase in file size and the two-fold increase in scan time required by a 5 μm scan. To check for yourself that 10 μm scans are adequate for features over 100 μm in diameter, scan the same slide, once at 5 μm and once at 10 μm, and divide the analyzed microarrays in Axon Instruments' Acuity™ microarray informatics software, or in Microsoft Excel, and observe that the spot ratios are the same at both resolutions.

5.6.2 Key Graphical Tools

5.6.2.1 Ratio Image

What biological information is conveyed by a ratio image? The ratio image typically represents the level of test to reference cDNA that is hybridized to spotted (or arrayed) cDNA. Suppose the reference cDNA is labeled with Cy3 (which is excited by green laser light such as 532 nm), and suppose the test cDNA is prepared in the presence of Cy5 (which is excited by red laser light such as 635 nm). Both of these cDNA populations are hybridized to the spotted cDNA on a microscope slide. In the derived ratio image, a red spot indicates that the test cDNA for this feature is more abundant than the reference cDNA, which means that it is being expressed at a level higher than the reference. A green spot indicates that the test cDNA is being expressed at a level lower than the reference cDNA; a yellow spot means that there is no change in the expression level between the two populations of test and reference cDNA. A ratio image should therefore provide a visual summary of the expression levels on the whole microarray.

The other use of a ratio image is as a quick way of estimating the microarray's quality. Large-scale defects, such as smears, or systematic spotting problems, such as missing or damaged pins, are most easily diagnosed by inspection of the ratio image.

5.6.2.2 Scatter Plot

Scatter plots convey a similar amount of information as ratio images. Whereas a ratio image displays expression levels by color, a scatter plot displays them as a distance from the diagonal on a graph. The GenePix Pro software employs two different types of scatter plots. The first, known as the Feature Pixel Plot, plots pixel intensities from individual features, so that one can evaluate the quality of the data from individual spots of DNA.

The second, on the Scatter Plot tab, allows one to plot any extracted data quantity from the whole microarray against any other, so for example one can plot mean intensities at the first wavelength against mean intensities at the second wavelength, or medians against medians, or raw pixel intensities against raw pixel intensities. Among the more useful scatter plots are:

• *Red intensity vs. green intensity*: the diagonal through the origin separates features with a higher activity than the reference from features with a lower activity than the reference. If the data cloud lies significantly off the 45-degree diagonal, it may indicate a significant difference in channel intensity that should be normalized.

• *Spot number vs. ratio*: the chosen ratio is displayed as greater or less than 1.0 for all spots. Differentially regulated features are more easily identified than on a standard intensity comparison plot.

• *Sum of medians (log axis) vs. log ratio*: highlights low intensity spots with artificially high ratios. If the denominator of a ratio is very low, the resulting ratio value may be artificially high. You can use this plot to identify such false outliers.

5.7 Normalization

There are close to as many normalization methods as there are people using microarrays. One of the reasons for this is that there is no agreement on the meaning of 'normalization', and so many different types of numerical manipulation are placed under this broad term. A second reason is that there are many different systematic defects with microarray data, each of which can be corrected with a different numerical method. Ochs and Bidaut discuss the topic in detail in Chapter 7 of this book. We will briefly outline some approaches to numerical manipulation.

5.7.1 Types of Numerical Manipulation

The many different types of numerical manipulation that can be applied to microarray data can be divided into two groups:

Data correction: alters experimental data to correct a systematic experimental error. Data correction is only acceptable when the systematic error is known and well characterized, and when it is a short cut to performing the experiment again with the systematic error removed from the procedure. The corrected values are the true values, free of systematic error.

Data pre-processing: removes data points and standardizes the distribution of the data so that we can compare multiple experiments, or so that the data is in an acceptable format for downstream analysis such as clustering.

5.7.2 Data Correction

The most common reason for performing data correction in microarray experiments is to correct for a scanner with an uncalibrated ratio channel. For a data distribution in which the average ratio value is different from 1.0, we can scale the intensity data in each channel with a linear transformation so that the ratio is equal to 1.0. Since PMT response is linear over a wide range of incident light, this type of data correction is equivalent to performing the experiment again with the PMT's calibrated. The linear transformation matches the instrument adjustments, and so we are justified in correcting the data.

Nevertheless, if the ratio across the whole slide is significantly different from 1.0 (say, more than 1.25 or less than 0.8) it is recommended that you do scan the slide again with the PMT's calibrated.

The same linear scaling of the data is acceptable where one considers a subset of spots on the array, for example a set of normalization or control spots. If the control spots have been chosen so that we can expect their median ratio to be 1.0, but the ratio is different from 1.0 because of our scanner's PMT settings, we can apply a linear normalization factor and scale the data from the whole slide so that the ratio of the control spots is 1.0.

A linear transformation to correct the balance between red and green across a whole slide is one method of normalization. There are a number of non-linear transformations that are also used to correct microarray data. A non-linear transformation corrects different spot intensities differently, so that, for example, low intensity spots are shifted differently to high intensity spots. These transformations are popular because if we do a scatter plot of red intensity versus green intensity, we often see the lower part of the scatter plot curving towards the red or the green, when we expect a straight line through the origin. A linear transformation shifts the distribution up or down without changing its shape; a non-linear transformation changes the shape of the distribution.

One of the more common non-linear normalization methods used on microarray data is Lowess (locally weighted scatter plot smoothing), championed by Dudoit et al.[3]. What imbalances in the data does Lowess normalization correct for?

Reasons for the imbalance in the two channels include properties of the dyes themselves (e.g. different labeling efficiencies and scanning properties) and experimental variability resulting, for example, from separate reverse transcription and labeling of the two samples.[4]

Lowess normalization is problematic because the defects in experimental design or execution that are being corrected are not sufficiently well understood. There is no mathematical model of "the properties of the dyes" or their "labeling efficiencies" analogous to the mathematical model of the response of PMT's at different intensities. Therefore we recommend caution when using Lowess normalization.

Whether or not you use Lowess normalization will depend on your attitude towards the use of statistical techniques for data correction. Statistical techniques like Lowess normalization can be used in one of two ways: to diagnose problems with experimental design and execution, or to correct those problems in software. If you are considering using Lowess normalization, you need to ask yourself:

a) Do I understand the physical basis of the defects that I am correcting?

b) Could I perform this experiment with its systematic errors corrected and obtain the same results as I get from the Lowess normalization of an experiment that has not had its systematic errors corrected?

If the answer to either of these questions is 'No', then it would be wiser to perfect your experimental technique to remove intensity-specific artifacts, than to modify your data without clearly understanding the reasons for the modification. If you do not understand the physical basis of what you are correcting, then you can have no more confidence in the corrected data than in the uncorrected data.

5.7.3   Data Pre-Processing

Pre-processing is applied to raw microarray data before further analysis operations. There are two basic types of pre-processing: removing sets of spots based on quality control criteria, and standardizing the distribution of data so that data from multiple microarrays can be compared.

To remove spots based on quality control criteria you need to translate general spot properties into mathematical conditions on your microarray data.

ensures the image collected is an accurate representation of the fluorescent sample. Key considerations include instrument calibration, detection limits, signal-to-noise ratio, dynamic range, and image resolution. Ratio image display and scatter plots aid immediate interpretation of the results, while additional analytical operations such as normalization, transformation, centering and scaling prepare data for the extensive cluster analysis that can reveal the complex biological interactions in large-scale experiments.

References

1. *DeRisi JL, Iyer VR, Brown PO*: Exploring the metabolic and genetic control of gene expression on a genomic scale. *Science* 1997;278:211-287.

2. *Basarsky T, Verdnik D, Wellis D, and Zhai J*: An overview of a DNA microarray scanner: design essentials for an integrated acquisition and analysis platform; in Schena M (ed): Microarray Biochip Technology. *BioTechniques Books*, Eaton Publishing, 2000.

3. *Pickett S, Basarsky T, Verdnik D, Wellis D*: Microarray scanning and data acquisition; in Geschwind DH, Gregg JP (eds) Microarrays for the Neurosciences: An Essential Guide. *MIT Press*, Cambridge MA, 2002.

4. *Dudoit S, Yang YH, Callow MJ, and Speed TP*: Statistical methods for identifying differentially expressed genes in replicated cDNA microarray experiments; *University of Berkeley Technical Report # 578*, August 2000.

CHAPTER

MICROARRAY IMAGE PROCESSING AND QUALITY CONTROL

Anton Petrov, Shishir Shah, Sorin Draghici *and* Soheil Shams

Contact:
Soheil Shams, Ph.D

BioDiscovery, Inc., 4640 Admiralty Way, Suite 710, Marina del Rey, CA 90292, U.S.A.
E-mail: sshams@biodiscovery.com

0-9664027-5-8/02/$0.00+$.50   *From:* **Microarray Image Analysis-Nuts & Bolts** (pp.99-130)
©2002 by DNA Press, LLC   Edited by: S. Shah and G. Kamberova

6.1 Introduction

DNA and protein array experiments, which employ printing of biological material on solid surface and consequent hybridization, require the ability to manage large quantities of data both prior to and following the actual experiment. There are three major issues involved in data management[1]. The first is to keep track of the information generated at the stages of chip production and hybridization steps[2]. The second is to analyze microarray images and to obtain the quantified gene expression values from the arrays. The third is to mine the information from the gene expression data[3]. The objective of this chapter is to discuss image segmentation and quality control issues related to array image analysis.

The goal of array image processing is to measure the intensity of the spots of printed biological material, quantify gene expression values based on these intensities, assess the reliability of the data, and generate warnings to the possible problems during the array production and/or hybridization phases. Microarray images consist of arrays of spots arranged in sub-grids, that are also called sub-arrays or quadrants (Figure 6-1). All the sub-grids usually have the same numbers of rows and columns of spots. These sub-grids are arranged in relatively equal spacing with each other, forming a "meta-array".

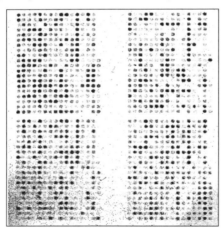

Figure 6-1. The image consists of four sub-arrays. It was printed by four pins (2x2). Each sub-array has the same number of rows and colums of spots, i.e. 20x16 respectively.

Ideally, a simple computer program could easily accomplish the image-processing task by superimposing an array of circles with defined dimensions and spacing on the images. In theory, the pixels falling inside and outside these circles would be considered signal and background, correspondingly. In reality, however, the exact location of each sub-grid may vary from slide to slide. There is a number of sources contributing to the problems, mainly due to mechanical constraints in the spotting process, hybridization inconsistencies, and the necessity to spot dense arrays to increase the efficiency of hybridization experiments. The problem of inconsistent spot location necessitates a reliable approach for automatic spot finding.

One of the primary concerns in reliable quantification of RNA expression values is the maximization of signal-to-noise ratio (SNR) in the raw image[4,5]. This quantity signifies how well one can resolve a true signal from the noise in the system. The SNR within an image can be estimated by computing the peak signal divided by the variation in the signal. If the scanning system generating the image has poor SNR, an accurate quantification of individual spots becomes very difficult. We characterize and model all imaging systems as linear and hence noise characterization is implicit in the process. Knowing the functionalities of a particular imaging system can help in improving the SNR, thereby aid in performing accurate analysis of the signal. As the image is a function of the incident light or photons, a photomultiplier tube is used to detect the photons and quantize the value to report intensities in an image. Due to thermal emissions and current leakage, electronic noise is introduced in the system. Such a noise can typically be modeled as Gaussian distributed white noise. The amount of this noise in the image can be reduced by controlling exposure time and gain while scanning.

The second noise type introduced in the system is related to number of incident photons. Due to the natural distribution of photons, as the number of incident photons is increased, the variability in its number also increases. Thus, as the intensity increases, the noise also increases. This variability is proportional to the square root of the signal.

The third source of noise that is important for image analysis is not dependent on the imaging system. The substrate of the slide can have large effects in the signal-to-noise ratio. The substrate material used can contribute towards background fluorescence, which will reduce the sensitivity of the signal. Improper treatment of the slide surface will result in poor attachment of the DNA, and hence reduce the resultant signal. Finally, residual material and improper handling and drying of the slide will result in background fluorescence.

Contamination is also a major source of problems in the microarray image processing. From the procedure of spotting to hybridization experiments, dust floating in the air may land on the slides and they are often very bright in the scanned images. Certain drying rates may cause little "bumps" in the spot surface, producing specular reflections in the images. Contamination may also come from splashes and drips of DNA solution from pins or impurities in the sur-

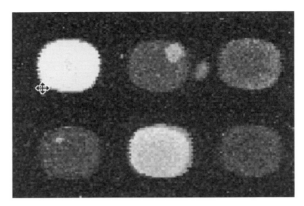

Figure 6-2. Contamination in microarray images is present in both background and inside of the spots.

face. Figure 6-2 shows an example of contaminations in a microarray image. Small contamination spots distributed in the background and the small contamination particles inside the spots with extreme intensity level are well noticed. The best solution to these problems is to identify the contamination and remove it before applying measurements.

The function of image processing is not limited to measuring the hybridization strength of each spot. One way or the other, detecting the problems in microarray images is indispensable for ensuring the validity of the data and improving the quality of chip production and experimental procedure. The information exchange needs to tie back with the array design and fabrication process, which can easily be done through a common underlying data management system.

6.2 Noise Suppression

The process of imaging is modeled as a linear system where the image is obtained as an output of the ideal signal convolved with the impulse response of the imaging system. Knowing the impulse response of the system and deconvolving the obtained image with it can achieve noise suppression or filtering. Due to complexity of the imaging process and the other factors degrading the quality of the image, modeling it as a linear system and hoping to find a perfect impulse response to that system is a rather simplistic view. In practice, one has to choose a filter based on an assumption of the noise process in the system[6]. Using linear filters may compromise the localization accuracy of the spots, thus they do not form an ideal choice even if the SNR improvement prove to be significant. An alternative approach is to use the median filter. One can perform one-dimensional or two-dimensional median filtering. In either case a window configuration should be pre-set. The window is usually centered at the current pixel and covers some neighborhood. The pixel value then is replaced with the median computed over this window. After that the window is moved and centered at the next pixel. This is an effective nonlinear filter, which removes impulse and "salt and pepper" noise while retaining details.

A useful variation on the theme of the median filter is the *percentile filter*, where the center pixel in the window is replaced not by the 50% (median) brightness value but rather by the *p%* brightness value where *p%* ranges from 0% (the *minimum filter*) to 100% (the *maximum filter*). In an effort to preserve details within the image while reducing the noise, edge-preserving filters also form a good choice. The Kuwahara filter replaces the pixel value with the mean value of the local neighborhood region that has the smallest variance. This would aid in preserving the mean signal and background values while removing impulse noise.

6.3 Spot Finding Methods for Resolving the Spot Localization Errors

The goal of spot finding operation is to locate the signal spots in images and estimate size of each spot. There are three different levels of sophistication in the algorithms for spot finding, corresponding to the degree of human intervention in the process. These are described below in order most to least amount of manual intervention.

6.3.1 Manual Spot Finding

This method is essentially a computer-aided image processing approach. The computer itself does not have any visual capabilities to "see" the spots. It provides tools, which allow the users to tell the computer where each of the signal spots is in the image. Typically, a grid frame is given that the user can manually place on the image and manipulate the grid frame to fit to the spatial extent of the spots in the image. Because the spots in the image may not be evenly spaced, the user may need to adjust the grid lines individually to align with the arrayed spots. The user may also have to adjust some grid points to land onto the spots in the image. The size of each circle may also need manual adjustment to fit to the size of each particular spot. To conduct an accurate measurement, this method is prohibitively time-consuming and labor intensive for images that have thousands of spots. Considerable inaccuracy of the data may be introduced due to human errors, particularly with arrays having irregular spacing between the spots and large variation in spot sizes. Historically, this was the first method of choice for microarray image analysis available through share software packages developed by academic institutions such as Stanford

University, National Institute of Health, and others in the early days of this novel technology for high throughput screening for gene expression levels.

6.3.2 Semi-Automatic Spot Finding

The semi-automatic method requires some level of user interaction with the software in terms of "instructing" where to place the grids of circles and how to find the spots on an image. This approach typically uses algorithms for automatically adjusting the location of the grid lines, or individual grid points after the user has specified the approximate location of the grid. What the user needs to do is to tell the program where the outline of the grid is in the image. For example, the user may need to put down a grid and adjust the size of it to fit on the array of the spots, or to tell the program the location of the corners of the sub-grids in the images (Panel 6-A). Then the spot finding algorithm adjusts the location of the grid lines, or grid points, to locate the arrayed spots in the image. User interface tools are usually provided by the software to allow for manual adjustment of the grid points in the event of a failure for the automatic spot finding method to correctly identify each spot.

This approach could potentially offer great timesaving over the manual spot finding method since the user needs only to identify a few points in the image and make minor adjustments to a few spot locations if required.

The key issue for spot finding algorithms here is to correctly identify the spots even at very low levels of intensity. In addition, the algorithm must deal effectively with two opposing criteria. First, due to variation in spot position, as described earlier, the algorithm must tolerate a certain degree of irregularity in the spot spacing. At the same time, the algorithm must not be distracted by contaminants that could be adjacent to a true arrayed spot. Panel 6-B outlines a practical strategy for dealing with such problems.

6.3.3 Automatic Spot Finding

The ultimate goal of array image processing is to build an automatic system, which utilizes advanced computer vision algorithms, to find the spots without the need for any human intervention. This method would greatly reduce the human effort, minimize the potential for human error, and offer high consistency in the quality of data. Such a processing system would require the user to only specify the expected configuration of the array (e.g., number of rows and columns of spots). The system would automatically search the image for the grid position. Most of the methods used for this purpose are based on some type of matched filtering. Matched filtering can be applied row- or column-wise or for the whole grid.

Having found the approximate grid position, which specify the centers of each spot, the neighborhood can be examined for signal and background regions. Knowledge about the image characteristics should be incorporated to account for variability in microarray images. Assumptions about the spot location, size, and shape should be adjusted to accommodate for noise, contamination and uneven distribution. Panel 6-C outlines a procedure for complete automated microarray image analysis. This approach is unbiased and yields high quality data. Human intervention and possibilities for errors are minimized.

6.4 Spatial Segmentation of Signal and Background Pixels

After the spot location is determined in the image, a small patch around that location (target region) can be used to quantify the spot expression level. A patch or a snip is a rectangular area around the spot, in which the signal and background pixel values are measured. The next step is to determine which pixels in the target region are due to the actual spot signal and which are background, a procedure known as image segmentation[7]. At this stage, the size and shape irregularities of the spots and any contamination problem in the images are the major concern to the algorithm design. A number of methods have been developed with different levels of sophistication.

6.4.1 Pure Space Based Image Segmentation

Methods of this class, known also as fixed circle segmentation, use purely spatial information from the result of spot finding to segment out signal pixels. After the spot finding operation has been completed, the location and size of the spot is determined. A circular mask of the computed size is placed in the image at the determined position to separate the signal from the background. It is assumed that the pixels inside the circle are correspond to the true signal and those outside are background. Measurements are then performed on these classified pixels.

These types of methods are optimal when the spot finding operation is effective, i.e., spots have been correctly located and sized, the spot shapes are close to perfect circles, and no contamination is present[8]. Knowing the configuration of the array and the spacing between spots, the user can specify the number of pixels around the spot that can be used to estimate the background intensity. However, irregularity of the spot shape and sizes are more like rules than exception in microarray images. Whenever these conditions occur, the accuracy of the measurements is largely compromised. In addition, spot contamination is still present in many microarray images. In the real life, a pure spatially based segmentation although being computationally inexpensive on one hand, becomes critically inaccurate on another hand (Figure 6-3).

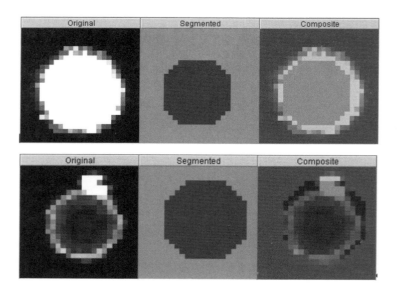

Figure 6-3. Circular (pure spatial) segmentation results from a two-dye experiment. There is contamination in the second channel (bottom row), which is not handled well by this type of segmentation. The pixels that are due to the contamination will be counted as part of the background in this case.

6.4.2 Pure Intensity Based Signal Segmentation

Methods of this class use intensity information exclusively to segment out signal pixels from the background. They assume that the signal pixels are statistically brighter than the background pixels. As an example, suppose that the target region around the spot taken from the image consists of 40x40 pixels. The spot is about 20 pixels in diameter. Thus, from the total of 1600 (40x40) pixels in the region, about 314 (πx10^2) pixels, or 20%, are signal pixels and they are expected to have higher intensity than that of the background pixels. To identify these signal pixels, all the pixels from the target region are ordered in a one dimensional array from the lowest intensity to the highest one, $\{p_1, p_2, p_3,...,p_{1600}\}$, where p_i is the intensity value of the pixel of the i-th lowest intensity among all the pixels. If there is no contamination in the target region, the top 20% pixels in the intensity rank may be classified as the signal pixels. The advantage of this method is its simplicity and speed; it is good for obtaining results using computers of moderate computing speed. The method works well for clean, good, and contrast images. However, it has disadvantages when dealing with noisy, contaminated images of low contrast with spots of low intensities, negative expressions, or noisy images.

6.4.3 Mann-Whitney Segmentation

Based on the result of the spot finding operation, a circle is placed in the target region to include the spatial region of the spot. Because the pixels outside of the circle are assumed to be the background, the statistic properties of these background pixels can be used to determine which pixels inside the circle are signal pixels. Mann-Whitney test is used to obtain a threshold intensity level[9, 10].

Mann-Whitney segmentation can be done as follows. Randomly select some number of pixels from the background (say, 10 pixels), their intensity values will form the first sample. Select same number of signal pixels (again, 10 pixels), but choose those that have the lowest intensity values within the signal mask. Test the two samples for having the same means using Mann-Whitney test. If the samples pass the test, replace some pre-defined number of pixels from the signal sample with those not yet in the sample and having lowest intensity values. Testing will continue until two samples fail the test. Pixels inside of the circle with higher than the minimal intensity of the signal sample are identified as signal.

This method works very well when the spot location is found correctly and there is no contamination in the image. However, when contamination pixels exist inside of the circle, they will be determined as signal pixels. This is due to the fact that typical contamination will be seen as specular reflection and has intensity higher than the background. If there are contamination pixels outside of the circle, or the spot location is not found correctly, such that some of the signal pixels are outside of the circle, these high intensity pixels will raise the intensity threshold level. Consequently, the signal pixels with their intensity lower than the threshold will be misclassified as background. This method also has its limitations when dealing with weak signal and noisy images. When the intensity distribution functions of the signal and background are largely overlapping with each other, classifying pixels based on an intensity threshold is prone to classification errors, resulting in measurement biases. This scenario is similar to what has been discussed in the pure intensity based segmentation method.

6.4.4 The Method of Trimmed Measurements

The trimmed measurements approach combines both spatial and intensity information in segmenting the signal pixels from the background. The logic of this method proceeds as follow. After the spot is localized and a circle is placed in the target region, most of the pixels inside of the circle are signal pixels and most of the background pixels are outside of the circle. Due to the shape irregularity, some signal pixels may leak out of the circle and some background pixels may get into the circle. These pixels may be considered as outliers in the samples of the signal and background pixels. Similarly, contamination pixels may also be considered as outliers in the intensity domain. These outliers will severely change the measurement of the mean and total signal intensity. To remove the effect of outliers on these measurements, one may simply "trim-off" a fixed percentage of pixels from the intensity distribution of the pixels for both signal and background regions (Figure 6-4). However, one never knows *a priori* what outlier percentage would be "right" for a spot and again, such an approach can produce inaccurate results.

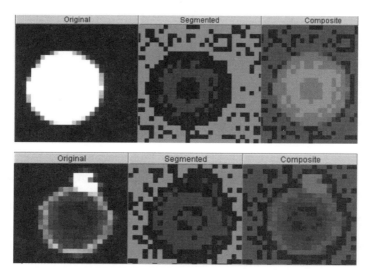

Figure 6-4. Results of "trimmed measurements" segmentation.

6.4.5 Integrating Spatial and Intensity Information for Signal Segmentation

The Mann-Whitney test and the method of trimmed measurements dis-cussed above use minimal amount of spatial information, i.e. the target circle obtained from spot localization is not used to improve the detection of signal pixels. Their design priority is to make the measurements of the intensity of the spots with minimal computation. These methods are useful in semi-automatic image processing because the speed has strong priority and the user can visu-ally inspect the quality of the data.

In a fully automated image processing system, the accuracy of the signal pixel classification becomes a central concern. Not only does the correct segmentation of signal pixels offer accurate measurement of the signal intensity, but it also permits multiple quality measurements based on the geometric properties of the spots. These quality measures can be used to draw the attention of a human inspector to spots having questionable quality values after the completion of an automated analysis (Figure 6-5). The correct classification of the signal pixels can be realized by algorithms that use information from both spatial and intensity domain (hybrid methods)[11,12,13, 14].

The microarray image segmentation procedure, which is based on the integration of the spatial and intensity-based approaches, can be divided into three stages.

• Initially, information about spot location and diameter is utilized by purely spatial (circular) segmentation.

• Subsequently, distribution outliers for inside and outside of the circle are defined as "undetermined" pixels. Gaussian model for intensity distribution is usually used for outlier detection.

• During the final stage, re-labeling of "undetermined" pixels as "signal", "background" or "contamination" occurs. This re-labeling is based on region growing procedure. Region growing will re-label every "undetermined" pixel according to the results of a statistical test against neighboring background and signal pixels. Region growing should be applied iteratively until no re-labeling can be performed.

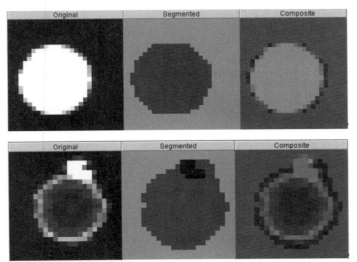

Figure 6-5. Segmentation results of a "hybrid" method.

6.5 Data Quantification

Quantification is the process, which deals with the measuring of the spot signal and background values. The key information that needs to be recorded from microarrays is the expression strength of each target. In gene expression studies, one is typically interested in the difference in expression levels between the test and reference mRNA populations. This translates into differences in the function of intensities on the two images. Under idealized conditions, the total florescent intensity from a spot is proportional to the expression strength. These idealized conditions are:

• The preparation of the probe cDNA (through reverse transcription of the extracted mRNA) solution is done appropriately, such that the probe cDNA concentration in the solution is proportional to that in the tissue.

• The hybridization experiment is done appropriately, such that the amount of cDNA binding on the spots is proportional to the probe cDNA concentration in the solution.

• The amount of cDNA deposited on each spot during the chip fabrication is constant.

• There is no contamination on the spots.

• The signal pixels are correctly identified by the image analysis software.

In the following discussion, we assume that the first two conditions are satisfied. Whether these two conditions are truly satisfied should be controlled through the design of the experiments. For the measurement obtained based on image analysis algorithms, we are mainly concerned about the remaining three conditions. In most cases, last three conditions are violated. The DNA concentrations in the spotting procedure may vary from time to time and spot to spot. Higher concentrations may result in larger spot sizes. When contamination is on the spot, the signal intensity covered by the contaminated region is not measurable. The image processing may not correctly identify all the signal pixels, thus, the quantification methods should be designed to address these problems. The common parameters computed from the intensities of the detected signal pixels are total, mean, median, mode, volume, intensity ratio, and the correlation ratio across two channels. The underlying principle for judging which one is the best method is based on how well each of these measurements correlates to the amount of the DNA probe present at each spot location.

Total. The total signal intensity is the sum of the intensity values of all the pixels in the signal region. As it has been indicated above, the total intensity is sensitive to the variation of the amount of DNA deposited on the spot, the existence of contamination, and the anomalies in the image processing operation. Because these problems occur frequently, the estimated *total* may not be an accurate measurement.

Mean. The mean signal intensity is the average intensity of the signal pixels. This parameter has certain advantages over the *total*. Very often the spot size correlate to the DNA concentration in the wells during the spotting processing. Measuring the mean will reduce the error caused by the variation of the amount of DNA deposited on the spot. With advanced image processing allowing for accurate segmentation of contamination pixels from the signal pixels, the mean should be the best measurement method.

Median. The median of the signal intensity is the intensity value that splits the intensity distribution of the signal pixels in halves. The number of pixels with intensity above the median intensity is the same as those below it. Thus, this value is a landmark in the intensity distribution profile. The advantage of choosing this landmark as the measurement is due to its resistance to outliers. As has been discussed in the last section, contamination and problems in the image processing operation introduce outliers in the sample of identified signal pixels. The mean measurement is very vulnerable to these outliers. When the distribution profile is uni-modal, the median intensity value is very stable and it is close to the mean. In fact, if the distribution is symmetric, the median is equal to the mean. Thus, if the image processing operation is not sophisticated enough to ensure the correct identification of signal, background, and contamination pixels, *median* is a better estimate of the true signal intensity than the *mean*. An alternative to the median measurement is to use trimmed mean, as discussed earlier. The trimmed mean estimation is the mean of the sample after certain percentage of pixels have been trimmed from the tails of the signal sample.

Mode. The mode of the signal intensity is the "most-likely" intensity value and can be measured as the intensity level corresponding to the peak of the intensity histogram. It is also a landmark in the intensity distribution. Thus, it enjoys the same robustness against outliers offered by the median. The trade-off is that the mode becomes a biased estimate when the distribution is multi-modal. When the distribution is uni-modal and symmetric, mean, median, and mode estimates are equal. Often the difference between mode and median can be used as an indicator of the degree to which a distribution is multi-modal.

Volume. The volume of signal intensity is the sum of the signal intensity above the background intensity. It may be computed as

$$V = (\mu_{signal} - \mu_{background}) \times A_{signal}$$

Where A is the spot (signal) area and μ stands for the means of the signal and the background. This method adopts the argument that the observed signal intensity has an additive noise component due to the non-specific binding and this component is the same as that from the background. This argument may not be valid because the non-specific binding in the background is different from that in the spot. Perhaps a better way is to use "blank" spots for measuring the strength of non-specific binding inside spots. These blank spots have no DNA (during printing the samples contained the printing buffer only without any biological sample). In some experiments the intensity on the spots may be smaller than that of the background, indicating that the nature of non-specific binding is different between what is on the background and inside of the spots. To a larger extent, the background intensity should be used for quality control rather than for signal measurement.

Intensity ratio. If the hybridization experiments are done in two channels, then the intensity ratio between the channels might be the only quantified value of interest. This value will be insensitive to variations in the exact amount of DNA spotted since the ratio between the two channels is being measured. This ratio can be obtained from the mean, median, or mode estimates of the intensity measurement for each channel.

Correlation ratio. Another way of computing the ratio estimate is to perform correlation analysis across the corresponding pixels in two channels of the same slide. The ratio between the pixels in two channels is computed by fitting a straight line through a scatter plot of intensities of individual pixels. This line must pass through the origin and the slope of it is the intensity ratio between the two channels. This ratio is also known as regression ratio. The method may be effective when the signal intensity is much higher than the background intensity. The motivation behind using this method is to bypass the signal pixel identification process. However, for spots of moderate to low intensities, the background pixels may severely bias the ratio estimation of the signal towards the ratio of the background intensity. Then the advantage of applying this method becomes unclear and the procedure suffers the same complications encountered in the signal pixel identification methods discussed above. Thus its advantage over intensity ratio method may not be warranted. One remedy to this problem is to identify the signal pixels first before performing correlation analysis. Alternatively, one could identify the pixels that deviate within a specified amount from the mean of the intensity population.

Table 6-1 lists the results of mean, median, mode, and total quantification measurements using three signal pixel identification methods as applied to the image in Figure 6-5. In the case of the trimmed method, 30% of the signal pixels were trimmed from the low intensity side of the distribution and 20% from the high intensity side. For background pixel identification, pixels in a 3-pixel wide ring outside of the signal circle were discarded due to their potential of containing signal pixels "bleeding" into this region. In addition, 30% of the remaining background pixels were trimmed from the high intensity side. The measurements were done after the trimming. The combined intensity and spatial segmentation was used to identify signal, background, and contaminated pixels before computing the intensity measurement. The measurements were based on the segregated regions.

Table 6-1. Measurements using different quantification and image processing methods

	Mean	Median	Mode	Total
Combined	833.95	934.61	997.78	384450
Trimmed	1103.06	1109.42	1109.42	207375
Pure spatial	1232.80	1076.05	1063.25	464765

Because of the existence of contamination in the image, the mean method from the combined segmentation is optimal. The median and mode measurements are about 10-15% deviation from the mean. According to the trimmed method, the three measurements are very similar; and they are about 30% deviation from the mean of the combined technique. Without trimming, the mean measurement produces 50% deviation; however, median and mode estimations are essentially unchanged.

Based on our experience and observations, the mean is the best measurement when using the combined and trimmed segmentation techniques. Without trimming, median is the best choice. Although mode provides the same value as median in this case, in general it would be biased when the intensity distribution is multi-modal.

In estimating the true signal value, it is necessary to reduce the effect of nonspecific fluorescence, such as the auto-fluorescence of the glass slides. For most analysis calculations, the background intensity should be subtracted from the signal intensity before any ratio calculations are performed. The method for determining the background intensity can vary depending on the quality of the arrays and the spacing between individual spots. The same measurements discussed above, such as mean, median, mode, and total, can be used to compute the background. Further, one can also compute the standard deviation of the background intensities that can be used to determine the reliability of the measurement. If the standard deviation is high, the background is non-uniform and chances are that part of the signal is accounted for as background. If the spot spacing is too small, it may be advisable to compute a measurement value based on the grouping of several to all spots. The noise in the background region will ultimately determine how well one can resolve whether the signal is significantly above background. The noise is estimated by computing the standard deviation of the pixels in the background region. A common method for establishing signal threshold is to add one or two times the standard deviation to the background value. A spot with a measurement larger than this value is likely to be a true signal.

Quantification of overlapping spots presents a problem. This has been elegantly addressed by Brandle an colleagues[15]. A twist in their approach is that they use guide spots and hierarchical interpolation method based on Gaussian image pyramids. Their spot finding technique includes fitting of robust Gaussian spot models with the help of M-estimators, where the hybridization signal is determined as the volume of the analytic spot model.

6.6 Quality Measures

In a fully automated image processing system, the accuracy of the signal pixel classification becomes a central concern. Not only does the correct segmentation of signal pixels offer accurate measurement of the signal intensity, but it also permits multiple quality measurements based on the geometric properties of the spots. These quality measures can be used to draw the attention of a human inspector to spots having questionable quality values after the completion of an automated analysis. The correct classification of the signal pixels can be realized by algorithms that use information from both spatial and intensity domain.

There are currently several general approaches to expression quality measurement. Two different groups of methods can be noted in the literature.

• Image based quality assessment

• Replicate based quality assessment

Our current discussion will be mainly devoted to the first category, but in the beginning let us bring the other group under the scope for review purposes.

Spot replicates are considered to be a valuable source of information for significance and confidence analysis of differentially expressed genes[16].

However, they can also be successfully utilized for flagging of suspicious spots. The most common approach to quality control in this area is based on the replicate outlier removal. A presence of outlier replicate within expression distribution raises concerns about quality of the measurement. Algorithms of different complexities are currently available, however the most significant drawback of this approach is a necessity for fairly large number of replicates. Moreover, completely flawless replicate measurements would require quite complicated design of experiments.

Now, let us continue with the confidence measures assessed through a direct image analysis. Different quality measures can be used for such purpose; the choice of those mainly depends on a particular microarray design, equipment sophistication and measurement extraction procedures. The most widely used are the ratio of the signal standard deviation within the spot and its mean expression, the offset of the spot from its expected position in the grid and spot circularity measures (for example the ratio of a squared perimeter and a spot area.) These measures used separately, or combined into some kind of a decision tree can be used to flag a spot as of low quality. However it is not obvious how to compose a unique confidence number from such set of quantities.

Sources of spot expression miscalculation can be separated into two groups. The first group consists of measurement errors as consequences of defects introduced during slide printing and scanning process. The other group includes expression miscalculations following from poor performance of spot finding and image segmentation techniques applied to the image. In this chapter we will try to outline the set of rules one can use to account for the defects coming from both groups.

6.6.1 Background Contamination

A microarray image consists of one or several rectangular subgrids. The approximate structure of each subgrid, as well as the spacing between subgrids are usually known and are characterized by the type of printing and scanning hardware used in the experiment. Background defects may appear in arbitrary parts of an image due to various reasons. Such an artifact can influence the expression levels of a large number of spots located in the contaminated area. As mentioned earlier, we assume that the output of the segmentation procedure for each spot region delivers the signal (spot) pixels, background pixels around the spot and ignored pixels. The last ones are usually isolated from the rest of the image to avoid local contaminations (like dust particles) influencing the expression measurement. Our current task is to identify possible abnormality in the background.

Let us take the mean of the background intensity around the spot as the local background estimate. In an ideal situation, when no contamination occurs across the image, background means will be approximately normally distributed. A number of simple statistical tests can be applied to identify spots with significantly high or low background means. To illustrate our approach we used a standard t-test technique. All spot background means from an image are calculated. Subsequently, the average and the standard deviation of these background values are computed, and then the background mean of every spot is tested against these parameters with a t-test. A low p-value means that a contamination is present in the background of a spot.

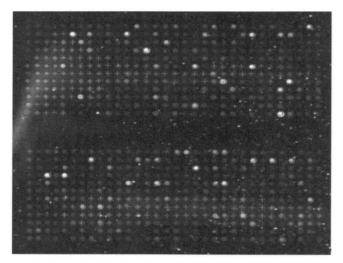

Figure 6-6. Background contamination flagging results. This image was processed using microarray software package ImaGene 4.2 (Biodiscovery, Marina del Rey, CA), where the aforementioned approach discussed in section 6.6.1 was implemented.

Figure 6-6 shows image of a slide with two subgrids 12x32 spots each (courtesy of The R.W. Johnson Pharmaceutical Research Institute, San Diego, CA). The circles bounding the spots have colors changing gradually from blue to red, red denoting the spots with a high contamination significance level. In other words, spots with the contaminated background have coloring shifted more to the red part of spectrum. The spots with contamination significance values greater than 95% are marked with "+". We can observe how the flags cover two suspicious regions, contaminated by bright traces in the background. Changing the threshold will be followed by changes in configuration of the flagged region. Lower threshold will produce more flags. This gathered information about the background can also be utilized for estimating the image- or sub-grid-wise background level and used for normalization.

6.6.2 Signal Contamination

Another possible source of signal disturbance can be a non-homogeneous distribution of material within the spot. To assess this quality we suggest to analyze a signal volatility within the spot. High signal variation will lower our confidence in the expression value. We suggest to take the spot intensity variance as an estimate of signal volatility. The spot intensity variance distribution can also be approximated by a normal distribution, however experiments show that the parameters of the distribution (its mean and variance) will strongly depend on the expression level of the spot. Thus, to retrieve more accurate information about signal variance distribution we collect all the spots on the image into groups by their expression levels. Then we sort the spots by the mean expression $\overline{X}_j$, and split them into bins with equal number of spots. And finally, we perform significance analysis similar to that described in the previous paragraph, but for each bin separately.

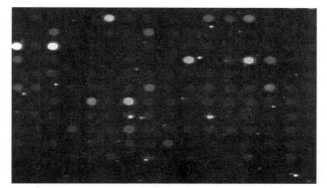

Fig 6-7. Signal contamination flagging results.

Figure 6-7 shows results produced by the microarray image analysis software ImaGene based on the signal contamination detection. The coloring scheme for the circles is analogous to that used in Figure 6-6 and the same threshold value was chosen. Bright contaminations occupying three spots on this image contribute to signal volatility within the spots, and as a result the corresponding spots are flagged out. There are some other spots in the image with significant level of contamination, however the image segmentation technique performs satisfactorily on those spots and contaminated pixels are ignored. One important issue that should be considered when we use this confidence number is the type of expression estimate (i.e. mean, median, mode, etc.) used per spot. If someone chooses the signal median or mode for his or her estimate of gene expression, such estimation procedure appears to be quite stable with respect to volatility of the signal and the threshold should be set at slightly higher levels than those used with the signal mean procedure.

6.6.3 Position Offset

The combination of the spot finding and image segmentation procedures give estimates for each spot's center location (for example, the center of mass of a spot region). To be able to test the results produced by this approach we should also obtain a co-called "expected position" of every spot in the grid. Obviously, for that purpose we could use locations of the nodes in a pre-defined rigid grid corresponding to idealistic microarray structure (see Panel 6-C). However, in real life many different factors can introduce systematic irregularities into the grid structure. Such irregularities as varying inter-row or inter-column distance or slight curvature in rows or columns should not influence our decision on spot quality. In such situation the best solution would be a least square fit of straight lines to the spot centers row- and column-wise. As a result, we can utilize intersection points of these lines as our expected spot locations. Once we obtain these coordinates, the testing procedure becomes relatively simple. We can compare the offset from expected position of every particular spot to an average expected inter-spot distance.

Flagging results received using ImaGene for offset analysis are shown on Figure 6-8. Settings we used for ImaGene were "flag every spot with an offset larger than 50% of average expected inter-spot distance". Flagged spots are located way off the grid positions and do not carry any meaningful measurements.

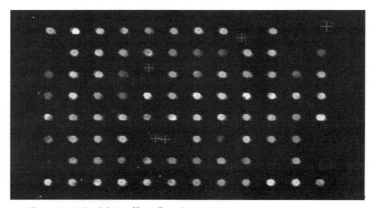

Figure 6-8. Position offset flagging results.

6.6.4 Percentage of Ignored Pixels

The signal contamination assessment we described previously does not take into the account any information about how many pixels were ignored during the segmentation procedure. Such information may give us additional understanding of the spot quality and may be extremely important if the ignored contamination region is attached to the signal area.

Let us compute the total number of pixels in the ignored regions that are directly neighboring the signal region for every spot. For each spot compute the ratio

$$R_j = \frac{\# \; of \; ignored \; pixels \; neighboring \; the \; signal}{\# \; of \; signal \; pixels \; + \; \# \; of \; ignored \; pixels \; neighboring \; the \; signal} \; x \; 100\%$$

For different microarray types different values of such a ratio might be acceptable. Thus set the threshold for flagging at some level R_0. Flag all the spots with the ratio higher than this threshold. Usually R_j below 10%-15% is acceptable.

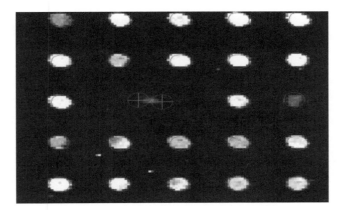

Figure 6-9. Ignored percentage flagging results.

ImaGene results show two flags in Figure 6-9, clearly indicating troubled spots. We set the threshold to 10%, however, this value should be chosen according to the microarray type. The threshold also should be chosen according to the researcher's tolerance to number of contaminated pixels. If for example, the user decides that 50% of the spot area are enough for reliable estimate, than the threshold should be adjusted respectively.

6.6.5 Percentage of Open Perimeter.

Sometimes the segmentation procedure isolates a wrong region as a signal. Usually this is the case when there is a contamination extended onto the territory of several spots. In such cases a signal region produced by the segmentation procedure frequently has a deformed shape that directly touches the boundary of spot's snip. In this case we can compute the perimeter of the spot signal P_{total} and the length of that part of signal boundary that coincides with the spot's region bounding box (the box around the spot, in which the segmentation procedure was performed) P_{open}. The ratio

$$\tilde{R} = \frac{P_{open}}{P_{total}} \; x \; 100\%$$

will be a measure of the percentage of "open" perimeter of the spot signal. Set the threshold for flagging of the spot at some level $\tilde{R}_0$ Flag all the spots with the ratio higher than this threshold. Usually $\tilde{R}_j$ below 10% is acceptable, because it may be due to high spot density on a slide. But again, this threshold should be a subject to adjustment according to current experimental conditions.

6.6.6 Shape Regularity

Several measures can be used for estimating the goodness of the spot shape. One of them is the ratio of a spot area and its squared perimeter scaled by 4π. Such a measure seems natural since it is 1 for an ideal circle and any non-circular shape will have lower value. A different measure used in ImaGene for a similar purpose is the "shape regularity". This measure counts all the ignored and background pixels that fall within the circle fitted to the signal region. The result is the ratio of the number of those pixels to the area of the circle. This technique measures how deformed the actual signal region is with respect to the expected circular shape.

The aforementioned quantities can be separated into two groups:

• **Probabilistic:** background and signal contamination

• **Absolute:** position offset, percentage of ignored pixels, percentage of open perimeter, and shape regularity.

An advantage of the probabilistic approach is that it is adoptive to any particular microarray structure and image intensity level, and does not require any additional tuning. Another advantage is that we can just sum two quality measures with equal weights and use the result as a meaningful probability (just make sure that the sum of the weights is equal to 1). However the absolute measures described above are necessary as well. The spot should be flagged as of low quality whenever at least one of the tools produces a flag.

The number of confidence values used can be reduced if one believes that a specific type of contamination will never appear in particular experimental conditions or that it is not significant.

The statistical nature of the probabilistic measures is essential for detecting the targeted defects. If the statistical approach shown above is not used, one would have to adjust manually the thresholds for absolute measurements like background mean and signal standard deviation for every new image. Experiments with ImaGene proved that the outlined scheme provides a reliable detection of different types of defects. Our experiments showed performance that was superior to the manual flagging made by human operator. This effect comes from ability of the aforementioned statistics to detect slight abnormalities in spot measurements. Taking into account further sophisticated statistical analysis that is usually done on the obtained data, the elimination of such abnormalities may be of a significant value.

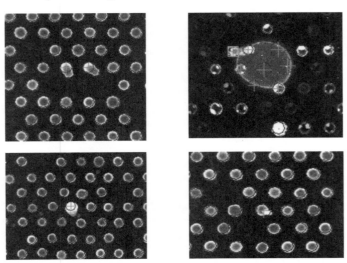

Figure 6-10. Various defects flagged by ImaGene version 4.2

6.7 Flagged Spots and Data Analysis

As we pointed out in the previous section, quality control in image analysis is important to guarantee that high quality data will be imported to the database and subsequently mined for expression patterns. The purpose of flagging individual spots is to identify those spotted samples the researcher desires to exclude from further analysis based upon quality parameters relating to the image segmentation pattern of the individual spots described earlier. These data are contained in a separate column in the output file from ImaGene named "Flag" and is expressed as a character code from 0-7 depending on the result. The character "0" designates spots having acceptable characteristics and the characters 1-7 indicate spots to be excluded due to automatic or manual flagging of empty, poor, and negative spots. As the case for all the data in an ImaGene file, the data are human readable using a standard text editor.

The BioDiscovery data mining and analysis software system GeneSight™ can directly read the flagged data and automatically exclude the designated spots from subsequent analysis. Moreover, GeneSight gives the researcher control over which category of flags are to be recognized. In GeneSight, the desired settings are entered using the Data Preparation facility, which is a GeneSight window containing drag-and-drop icons representing a variety of manipulations to be applied to the data such as background correction and normalizations. Applying a specific operation to the data is accomplished by creating a transformation sequence using icons for mathematical transformations of data. In the case of flags, selecting the "Omit Flagged Spots" icon and dropping it into the transformation sequence reveals a dialog box in which the analyst enters the ASCII character for the flag to be omitted. If spots flagged with differing ASCII characters are to be excluded, the researcher simply repeats the process dropping additional "Omit Flagged Spots" icons into the transformation sequence and entering the appropriate character in the dialog boxes. A researcher may want to omit spots that have been automatically flagged as "empty" from the analysis. Therefore, a numerical flag (in this case the number 2) needs to be entered in the appropriate window of the data mining system.

A key feature of GeneSight, which is important in evaluating the consequences of omitting flagged spots, is the ability to visualize the effects of removing the spots on the data set. GeneSight provides a variety of data visualization tools such as scatter plots that can be set to depict the data in one channel as a function of the data in a second channel. Combining this feature with the data preparation feature mentioned above, the investigator could visualize any unusual trends in the flagged data by observing the effect of removing the data from flagged spots when the entire data set is presented as a scatter plot. For example, one would typically expect that the preponderance of spots to be excluded based on quality parameters also have relatively low fluorescence intensity. A deviation from this expected pattern would be easily identified using this approach.

Combining spot flagging capabilities with visualization tools provides a powerful yet easy approach for including spot quality data in the overall analysis of microarray data.

References

1. *Zhou Y-X, Kalocsai P, Chen J-Y, Shams S.*: Information processing issues and solutions associated with microarray technology; In Schena M. (ed): Microarray Biochip Technology. Natick, *BioTechniques Books*, 2000, pp 167-200.

2. *Kuklin A, Smith J*: Microarray Experimental Design and Databasing with CloneTracker DB, ed 2, Marina Del Rey, BioDiscovery, 2001.

3. *Hoff B, Kuklin A, Shams S.*: Gene expression pattern analysis with clustering in the data mining system GeneSight(tm). *BIOforum International* 2001; 5:35-37.

4. *Duda RO, Hart PE*: Pattern Classification and Scene Analysis. *J. Wiley*, 1973.

5. *Haralick R M*: Statistical and structural approaches to texture. Proceedings of IEEE 1979; 67:786-804.

6. *Shah S, Aggarwal JK*: A Bayesian Segmentation Framework for Textured Visual Images. Proceedings of Computer Society Conference on Computer Vision and Pattern Recognition 1997: 1014-1020.

7. *Pal NR, Pal SK*: A review on image segmentation techniques. Pattern Recognition 1993;26:1277-1294.

8. *Price K*: Image segmentation: A comment on studies in global and local histogram-guided relaxation algorithms. IEEE Trans. on *PAMI* 1984; 6(2):247-249.

9. *Chen Y, Dougherty ER, Bittner ML*: Ratio-based decisions and the quantitative analysis of cDNA microarray images. *J. BioMedical Optics* 1997; 2(4):364-374.

10. *Johnson RA, Wichern DA*: Applied Multivariate Statistical Analysis, *Prentice Hall*, 1998.

11. **Shah S, Aggarwal JK**: Multiple Feature Integration for Robust Object Localization. *Proceedings of Computer Society Conference on Computer Vision and Pattern Recognition* 1998; pp 765-771.

12. **Shah S, Aggarwal JK**: Object Recognition and Performance Bounds. In Del Bimbo A (ed): Lecture Notes in Computer Science: Image Analysis and Processing. *Springer Verlag*, 1997, pp 343-360.

13. **Spann M, Nieminen A**: Adaptive Gaussian weighted filtering for image segmentation. *Pattern Recognition Letters* 1988; 8:251-255.

14. **J. M. Beulieu and M. Goldberg**. Hierarchy in picture segmentation: A stepwise optimization approach. IEEE Trans. on *PAMI*, 1989, V11(2):150-163.

15. **Brandle N, Bischof H, Lapp H**: Robust DNA microarray image analysis. Submitted.

16. **Hilsenbeck SG, Friedrichs WE, Schiff R, O'Connell P, Hansen RK, Osborne CK, and Fuqua SAW**. Statistical Analysis of Array Expression Data as Applied to the Problem of Tamoxifen Resistance, *Journal of the National Cancer Institute*, 1999, V91(5):453-459.

17. **Jain AN, Tokuyasu TA, Snijders AM, Segraves R, Albertson DG, Pinkel D**: Fully automatic quantification of microarray image data. *Genome Research* 2002; 12:325-332.

18. **Kuklin A, Shams S, Shah S**: Automation in microarray image analysis. *JALA* 2000; 5:67-70.

Panel 6-A

Creating Sub- and Meta-Grids of Spot-finding Circles

Each pin from a microarray printing device (whether a hand-held or an automated robot) prints an array of spots called a quadrant, sub-array or a sub-grid. To extract data from these spots the user needs to create a sub-grid of circles, which will overlay the spots. All the sub-grids form a meta-grid in the microarray image. There are two major approaches for creating sub-grids and meta-grids of circles in various software. The first one is interactive and requires some operator's involvement, whereas the second one is completely automated. A researcher needs to decide what approach to use based on the quality of the array images and the spot finding algorithm.

Let us consider the creation of a grid when a user "guides" the software to place the grid of circles. The software needs the information how many rows and columns are present in one sub-grid. Additionally, the user needs to determine a range for the minimum and maximum diameter of the circles that can be placed over the spots because the software algorithm uses these guidelines to position the circle over the spot based on pixel intensities. To measure the approximate diameter of spots on the array, a researcher may use a Ruler tool, hold the mouse, click on the edge of one spot, drag across the spot over the diameter, release the mouse at the opposite edge of the spot (Figure 6-A1) and see the reported distance (i.e. spot diameter) in pixels. Repeat this procedure for several spots and decide on an approximate number for the minimum and maximum diameter boundaries.

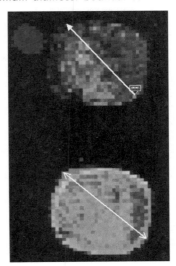

Figure 6-A1. The measurement of a spot diameter is achieved through a Ruler tool. A user identifies minimum and maximum spot diameter boundaries for, which guide the algorithm during the spot finding step.

Many users tend to give a broad range for the diameter. Note that this approach allows the software to create very large circles over spots, which have low expression values and contaminants in the background. This happens because the algorithm is "searching" for pixels with the highest values within the allowed parameters and if you assigned a lot of freedom in diameter size the circle expands and finds pixels with high intensities in the background. Since this is undesirable the users needs to decrease the maximum diameter. Note that depending on the image segmentation used, the user may not be concerned too much about "exact" placement of the circle over the spot.

After the approximate spot dimensions are determined and the number of rows and columns in one subgrid are registered, the user needs to guide the software during the creation of the first sub-grid. This is achieved by selecting the approximate center of the top-left corner spot, then connecting it with the top right corner spot, bottom right, and at the end, bottom left corner spot (Figure 6-A2). A sub-grid of spots is created automatically. You may save this sub-grid for future use. If you use the same array design you simply load the previously saved grid and in a second you are ready to run the image analysis.

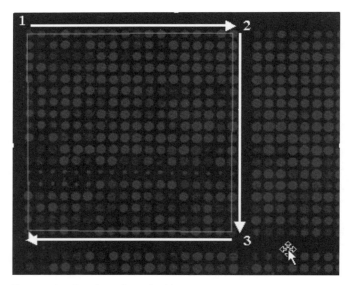

Figure 6-A2. Creation of a subgrid.

Microarray printing protocols in many laboratories worldwide require "staggered" printing pattern. This means that all even numbered rows of each sub-array are either indented to the right or extended to the left (Figure 6-A3).

Software, such as ImaGene usually have the option to accommodate such a printing pattern during the grid creation step.

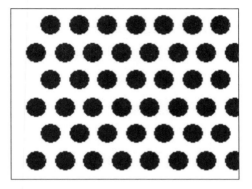

Figure 6-A3. A staggered spot pattern can be accomodated by the software during the sub-grid creation.

To create the meta-grid, the user needs to click on the top-left corner spot of each of the corner sub-grids in the meta-array. The software will automatically create the whole meta-grid. Most of the software will place the meta-grid of spot-finding circles automatically over the array of spots. If the intensities of the spots in some of the corners are very low, the user may need to position the grid of circles manually.

The second method for spot spacing and sub-array spacing requires only the geometry of of subarray grids and the geometry of spots in each sub-array[17, 18]. The user enters the number of rows and columns of spots in each sub-array and the number of rows and columns of sub-arrays in the whole array or meta-array. Estimation of spot and sub-array spacing is achieved automatically by summing the signal intensities in the X and Y directions of the image. The pattern of signal peaks is used to determine both the interspot spacing and the intersubarray spacing *(for detailed description consult with reference 17)*. This method may find difficulties in creating a meta-grid with poor quality array images.

Panel 6-B

Spot-Finding Procedures

The spots are expected to be printed in a regular geometric pattern so that the spot center overlays the crossing points (nodes) of a horizontal and vertical array of lines with equal spacing as corresponding to the difference between microplate wells (i.e. 4.5 mm for a 384 plate and 9 mm for 96 well plates) as shown in Figure 6-B1.

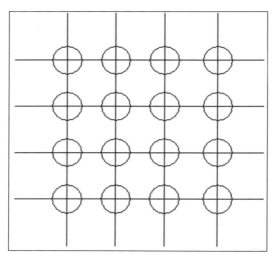

Figure 6-B1. Printed spots are ideally expected to be in a predetermined position. Their centers should be overlapping with the nodes of the horizontal and vertical lines.

However, misaligned arrayer pins or shaking of the arraying robot during printing may cause irregular printing pattern as shown in Figure 6-B2. In such a case, the spot finding circles can be given flexibility to go away from the theoretical centers of line crossing in the grid (Figure 6B-3) by a number of pixels that is empirically chosen by the user as shown in Figure 6B-4. The larger this number the greater the possibility for the circles to be affected by artifactual pixels in the background and deviate from the theoretical placement of the circle. Therefore, a user will usually find the best local grid flexibility for spot finding that suites the microarray image under analysis.

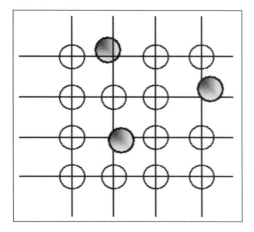

Figure 6-B2. In reality, there are always some spots that are not printed in the ideal positioned as shown in Figure 6-B1.

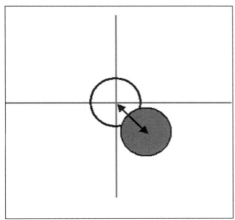

Figure 6-B3. A maximum distance in pixels between the expected theoretical spot center and the allowed deviation for the spot-finding circle may chosen by the user.

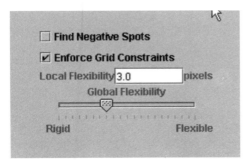

Figure 6-B4. A user can determine the flexibility for grid constraints.

Panel 6-C

Automation in Microarray Image Analysis

Recently the cDNA spotted microarray technology has proven to deliver more reliable results compared to the ones during first years of its development due to refined printing and hybridization protocols, as well as improved devices. This has prompted many researchers to use microarrays routinely and as a result the load of microarray images to be analyzed has been increasing drastically. The tremendous amount of generated images for various research and clinical trials projects has created a demand for automatic and unbiased strategy for microarray image analysis.

The images to be processed by the automated approach are loaded in a batch. The software needs an input of the gene IDs, the settings, and the destination folder for the analyzed data (Figure 6-C1). A gene ID file coupled with a grid is defined as a template. The configuration for a particular set of arrays is determined by the operator. The configuration file contains the settings for spot finding, image segmentation, and grid flexibility. A batch of arrays can consist of several array designs and corresponding configurations. The user can click the RUN button and walk away from the system. All processed data are deposited in a folder for subsequent analysis. The system provides a report, alert messages, segmented images of the processed microarray images, and a flat file with the quantified data through a ResultsReviewer™.

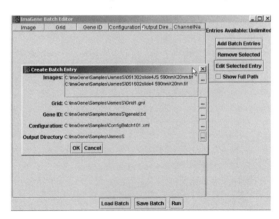

Figure 6-C1. All the images, template, configuration, and the folder for the results to be saved a determined through the batch analysis module.

Such an automated system is an invaluable tool for microarray core facilities because it brings unbiased processing of data and high quality of image analysis, which surpasses manual processing. Moreover, labor costs are drastically reduced and array data analysis between different labs and technology platforms is standardized for subsequent data analysis.

CHAPTER 7

MICROARRAY DATA NORMALIZATION

Michael F. Ochs[1] *and* Ghislain Bidaut[1,2]

1. *Department of Information Science and Technology, Fox Chase Cancer Center, Philadelphia*
2. *Structural and Genetic Information Laboratory, CRNS-AVENTIS, Marseille, France*

Contact:
Michael F. Ochs
Fox Chase Cancer Center, 7701 Burholme Avenue, Philadelphia, PA 19111 U.S.A.
E-mail: M_Ochs@fccc.edu

0-9664027-5-8/02/$0.00+$.50   *From:* **Microarray Image Analysis-Nuts & Bolts** (pp.131-154)
©2002 by DNA Press, LLC   Edited by: S. Shah and G. Kamberova

7.1 Background

7.1.1 Introduction

Gene expression microarrays are becoming ubiquitous in biological laboratories, with many academic institutions setting up facilities to produce arrays in-house. Biotechnology and pharmaceutical companies have produced numerous arrays either within their own research and development laboratories or through collaborations with specialized biotechnology companies, such as Rosetta Inpharmatics. These arrays provide a relatively inexpensive way to perform genome-wide measurements of gene expression under a variety of experimental conditions. However, to make use of these measurements, it is critical that proper and consistent data handling methodologies be applied. Normalization is a component of the required data handling and corrects for inconsistencies between the labeled cDNAs used in a microarray experiment, which arise from differences in labeling reactions, fluorescence properties of dyes, and other uncontrollable factors. This chapter discusses the issues of background correction and data normalization for microarrays probed with cDNA labeled with fluorescent dyes. Data normalization is also important for arrays labeled with radioactive probes, but may be more difficult in those cases[1].

7.1.2 Experimental Methods

As has been described in detail within this volume, microarrays consist of thousands of individual spots containing different DNA clones representing genes or ESTs derived from an organism of interest. The DNA spots are laid down on microscope slides, usually with treatment of the surface to increase binding of the DNA. Samples of mRNA are isolated from a control population and an experimental population, and these mRNA samples are reverse transcribed into cDNA probes. The labeling of the probes is either done directly with fluorescently labeled DNA bases that are inserted during reverse transcription or through inclusion of DNA bases with adapter molecules that allow attachment of fluorescent dyes after reverse transcription[2]. The control and experimental cDNAs are labeled with different dyes which fluoresce at different excitation frequencies (typically in the red and green segments of the visible spectrum). The microarray slides are then hybridized with an equimolar mix of the two labeled cDNA probes, often after a second pretreatment of the slide, this time to minimize nonspecific binding of the probes to the surface. After standard washes and other treatments, the slides are scanned in two passes (once at each excitation frequency), using a confocal laser scanner or other specialized system. The result is a set of two matched images, one for each of the two dyes representing the relative mRNA concentrations in the control and experimental samples. For the discussion below, it will be assumed that scanning was done in a manner to avoid saturation of the signal within any spot, excluding the possible saturation of small regions due to the presence of dust or other foreign material. The dynamic range of the measurements is scanner dependent, but is typically 16 bit, equivalent to 65535 to 1. If desired, multiple scans could be performed and the results merged to increase the dynamic range. If done appropriately this does not affect the normalization discussed below, but can complicate background correction.

7.1.3 Goals of Microarray Experiments

In order to determine how to handle microarray data normalization, it is important to understand the goals of the data generation and subsequent analysis. In a typical microarray experiment, a control population is defined (e.g. a cell line growing under standard conditions) and an experimental population linked to this control population is prepared (e.g. the same cell line growing under identical conditions but with the addition of a proposed therapeutic drug). The mRNAs of these populations are harvested using any of a number of standard protocols and used as templates for probe construction. The goal of the data generation and analysis in such a case is therefore a list of the genes that differ in expression between the two conditions[3-5]. More complex experiments, such as studies of genetic regulation through a biological process, may be performed as well[6-9], with the goal of understanding the patterns governing the changes of gene expression throughout a dynamic process. For both simple and complex applications, the need for correctly measured gene expression levels with minimal errors is critical, since with 5,000 to 40,000 genes typically being measured, error rates of even one percent will yield 50 to 400 false positives (i.e. genes which appear from the measurements to be differentially expressed but in reality are not). In addition, false negatives are expected as well, hiding true differential expression. While the multiple measurements performed during the exploration of a biological process may aid in reducing such false positives and negatives, it is unclear how errors feed into the pattern recognition process. Therefore the conservative approach dictates careful reduction of error prior to any analysis. These corrections must be done on a slide by slide basis, as they are generally slide dependent[10].

7.1.4 Sources of Errors in Measurements

Error enters the measurement of mRNA copy number in several ways. First, it must be noted that all measurements utilizing the two color fluorescently labeled cDNA method are measurements of the relative gene expression between the control and experimental populations, leading most researchers to report results as relative fold changes in the amount of mRNA for specific genes. The goal for data normalization is to insure that the intensity measurements made on the two images (control and experimental) are proportional to the mRNA concentrations. For this to be true, any systematic errors need to be correctly handled. These systematic errors arise from *1)* background fluorescence within the DNA spots on the array, *2)* false signals such as those due to fluorescence of dust within the spot, *3)* differences between the relative response to laser excitation of the two dyes used for control and experimental probes, *4)* differences in the incorporation efficiency of the dye-labeled bases during reverse transcription, and *5)* quenching effects that reduce the signal when the dyes fluoresce intensely (for a detailed discussion see[11]). In addition, there are errors which cannot be corrected for by data processing. These include most notably cross-hybridization of cDNA from genes having similar sequences and natural variation of expression unrelated to the experiment. The cross-hybridization problem is one of the driving forces behind the development of oligonucleotide arrays, where each oligonucleotide is designed for minimal cross-hybridization based on genomic sequence and EST databases[12]. The problem of natural variation is generally handled by replication of the experiment, preferably including full replication through all steps when possible, since even in well controlled yeast cultures there is substantial gene specific variation unrelated to a specific experimental protocol[13].

As noted above, there are multiple ways now available to label the cDNA that is hybridized to DNA spotted on the microarrays. The first method employed used cy3 or cy5 (fluorescent dyes) conjugated to dNTPs which were incorporated directly within the cDNA during reverse transcription from mRNA[9]. Because the dye molecules are large with significant size differences between them, they have different efficiencies in incorporation during labeling reactions, probably due to steric effects. As a result, one signal is generally significantly greater than the other signal following hybridization, not due to any inherent difference in mRNA concentration in the cells, but merely due to the incorporation differences. With new labeling methods using adapter molecules[2], the incorporation effects have been reduced. These adapter molecules contain a linker which, following reverse transcription of mRNA into cDNA, allows a fluorescent-probe labeled dendrimer to be attached. However, the linker approach does not solve all normalization problems. Even in experiments using the adapter labeling approach, additional normalization was required at the extremes of the intensity ranges in control experiments using the same sample labeled with two different dyes. The additional effects appear to be due to quenching of the signal at high intensity by reabsorption of the emitted light by the dye molecules[1], a process that is both intensity dependent and concentration dependent. The net result of the quenching is a reduction in signal at high intensity, leading to a requirement for nonlinear normalization.

Another problem in microarray measurements is that it is not clear that the background estimated from outside the DNA spots is representative of the background within the spots, which would make use of typical background corrections inappropriate (see below). This problem is probably not critical, as it appears that the overall noise in the measurements presently makes this a relatively small source of error. It has been noted that there appears to be both a multiplicative source of error, which relates linearly to the signal intensity, and an additive source of error due to background, such that the total error does not drop to zero as the intensity goes to zero[14]. If the background did not in some way contaminate the estimate of the intensity within the DNA spots, this would not be the case. Furthermore, the intensity related error makes a misestimation of the background (i.e. due to some difference between signal background and nonsignal background) less important at high intensity (i.e. high mRNA copy number), since the additive (i.e. background) error is less significant. As such, the most effected values are at low mRNA copy number, where most statistical analyses assume that the results are not significant[14-16].

7.1.5 Measurements for Data Processing

Images will be processed, as described elsewhere in this volume, to recover an estimate of the signal in each spot. Typically, three possible measurements are used: *1)* the mean value of all pixels which are considered signal, *2)* the median value of all pixels which are considered signal, or *3)* the total integrated intensity of all pixels which are considered signal. Presently all three methods are in use, with no clear indication in the literature demonstrating that one gives optimal results. In the discussion below, specific needs arising from methods of background correction and data normalization arising from the use of each of these measurements will be noted.

7.2 Background Correction

7.2.1 Sources of Background Intensity

Background correction is used to adjust the estimated signal during image analysis in order to remove signal unrelated to the specific binding of labeled cDNA probe to the matching DNA spotted on the microarray. This erroneous signal arises primarily from nonspecific hybridization and from intensity spikes, which result mostly from dust fluorescing highly under laser light. Figure 7-1 shows a detail of a microarray image with features marked. The two arrows point to spikes, one within a spot and one in the background region. Spikes within the spot are generally removed by thresholding, since scanning is typically done with the gain on the scanner adjusted to avoid saturation of real spots. Setting a threshold above which signal cannot be trusted will efficiently remove spikes. It is important to replace the signal removed with an estimate of the correct signal for that pixel if the mean value or integrated value of the intensity will be measured. For median measurements the loss of a single pixel should not significantly change the measurements, since typically there are over one hundred pixels in a spot region. Usually the adjoining pixels can be taken as an indicator of the correct value for a pixel removed in this way. Often a median rank filter or convolution filter can be used (see below for a discussion of these filters). Spikes outside the DNA spots are in the background portion of the image and are discussed below.

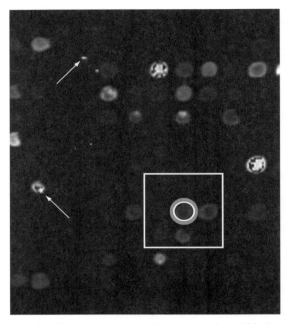

Figure 7-1. Schematic of a Microarray Image with Segmentation. This is an enlargement of a typical scanned microarray image in one channel (i.e. one color). The arrows show the presence of spikes of intensity caused either by dust or by some nonspecific binding of probe. The white circle shows the segmentation between signal (within the circle) and nonsignal for a single spot. Each spot on the array would have a similar circle or other shape separating signal from background. The shaded area represents the local background for the spot within the circle, while the white square represents a small neighborhood region around the spot.

A more difficult correction is for nonspecific hybridization. The expectation is that the nonspecific hybridization within a DNA spot is the same as the nonspecific hybridization outside a DNA spot. As noted above, this is not necessarily true[17], since the spotted areas of the array have had buffer from the solution containing DNA in contact with the surface, while surrounding areas have not. In addition, the use of different types of surface treatment on slides used for microarray production may lead to very different properties in the background. Keeping in mind this potential difference in background between spots and surrounding areas, the use of empty spots with buffer but lacking DNA spotted throughout the array should be used to monitor for this possible error. Throughout this chapter, it is assumed that overall the background within the spot is comparable to the signal outside the spot. However, if empty spots appear less intense than the background in a statistically meaningful way, an additional correction may be required.

7.2.2 Image Processing for Background Correction

It is useful to consider background correction as a specific application of image processing, which has a significant history with substantial tools that could be converted to use with microarrays[18, 19], including methods for background estimation[20]. In Figure 7-1 the segmentation of a single feature (i.e. a spot) on a microarray image into signal and local background is shown schematically. For each spot in the array, a similar separation can be made as described elsewhere in this volume, globally dividing the image into features (regions with signal) and background. In addition to a local region, larger regions can be defined on the image. The large white square represents one such possible region, called a neighborhood. Analysis of the behavior of images may be done on neighborhoods of any size, including one encompassing the entire image (i.e. global image analysis). In general, a neighborhood is taken to be a region comprising multiple features (i.e. spots). For the purpose of background estimation, the signal pixels are removed and operations are performed on the remaining pixels (i.e. background) only.

The estimation of the background for individual spots on an array can be viewed as a problem in image analysis, which can be addressed using one of three general approaches. The first approach is to use just the local background for each spot (as represented by the shaded portion of Figure 7-1). The use of a local background correction is justified by the patchiness in the nonspecific hybridization resulting from the hybridization step, which makes averaging over large areas prone to error[21]. The second approach is to use a local neighborhood of adjoining spots (such as within the white square in Figure 7-1). This is preferable to a local correction in most cases, since the patchiness in the background is usually larger than the size of a single spot. Sampling more of the image thus provides a more reliable estimate of the background intensity. The third approach is to perform a global analysis of the background, modeling the full background with an appropriate mathematical function. Usually this method is not used, since the background is generally known to be irregular, requiring a complex mathematical function for fitting. Such a function would be prone to local instabilities, thus removing the goal of estimating a smooth background and returning to a local correction, but with much greater computational cost. This last approach is not discussed further.

7.2.3 Local Background Correction

Local background correction uses a value calculated only within an area roughly the size of the shaded donut of Figure 7-1 and subtracts this from each pixel in the signal area (within the white circle). The value used can be either the median value or mean value of the background pixels. In general, a median value is considered a more reliable background estimator, since it is not prone to misestimation due to spikes or dropped pixels (i.e. pixels with no signal, either due to a scanning error or an image processing artifact). If a mean value is used, pixels with spikes must be removed and their intensity estimated. While widely used, a local background correction is probably not the best estimator, as a neighborhood analysis will analyze a larger region and provide a more reliable estimate.

7.2.4 Neighborhood Background Correction

Among possible neighborhood operations, three types appear suitable for consideration for background correction (as discussed in greater detail below). The first is a convolution filter, which analyzes the neighborhood of a spot and determines the best background estimator by performing a weighted average of the pixels in the neighborhood. Generally, background pixels nearer the signal pixel undergoing correction are given a greater weight than those near the edge of the neighborhood (white box in Figure 7-1). The second is a rank filter, which explores overall behavior in the neighborhood and chooses a value to apply. A background median filter, which calculates the median value in the background pixels in the neighborhood and subtracts it from each signal pixel, is a simple example of a rank filter. The third is an adaptive filter, which is designed to use properties of the features to determine what type of filtering to apply at each point. This is the most complex type of filter, but it provides more power if one can model the behavior of the image to some degree (e.g. areas with background patchiness can be treated differently than smoother areas).

7.2.4.1 Convolution Filters

Convolution filters, also called linear shift-invariant (LSI) filters, perform a mathematical operation using a point spread function (PSF) that defines how the filter responds to a point source (see Figure 7-2a). A PSF has an integrated value of 1 over the full function, which guarantees that the total intensity in an image after convolution is unchanged. For each pixel in the image, the

PSF is centered on the pixel and a new pixel value is calculated by summing over all pixels covered by the PSF. The sum is obtained over the product of the value of the PSF at each pixel and the pixel intensity. As a simple example of the effect of this operation, figure 2b shows two point sources, which are convolved with the PSF of Figure 7-2a, to yield Figure 7-2b. The effect of the convolution is to spread the intensity from the point sources over a wider range and bleed nearby points together.

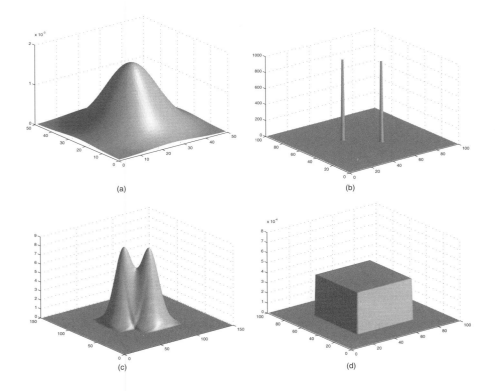

Figure 7-2. An example of a simple point spread function (PSF). *(a)* A Gaussian PSF is shown, which is used in the convolution for (c). *(b)* This simple image has two features that are spikes of intensity on an otherwise blank image. *(c)* Convolution of the PSF in (a) with the image in (b) results in this smoothed image. *(d)* The PSF shown represents the application of a mean filter on the neighborhood region of Figure 7-1.

Figure 7-3a is an unprocessed image, which is used to demonstrate how filtering affects images. Figure 7-3b shows the same image, but with the addition of spikes and Gaussian noise. In Figure 7-3c, the effect of a convolution with a Gaussian PSF is shown, indicating that a convolution generally smooths an image, potentially removing imperfections but causing a possible loss of resolution. The smoothing behavior makes convolution functions useful, since they can improve image interpretability if an image is reasonably uniform. They are, however, prone to errors when individual pixels of high intensity (such as spikes) appear within the neighborhood of the pixel under examination. The convolution function in this case will replace the individual pixel value with a value derived in part from the large intensity of the spike. One of the problematic issues which arise with convolution filters is the fact that they treat all pixels as reliable estimates of the physical system. For this reason, removing spikes prior to application of a convolution filter is necessary with microarray data, since otherwise the background is overestimated due to contamination from the spikes. Even a simple version of the convolution filter, a mean filter, which takes the mean value of a neighborhood region as the estimation of the background, requires removal of spikes prior to application. The mean filter is equivalent to a flat PSF, shown in Figure 7-2d. This type of filter has been applied as part of the segmentation process as well[22].

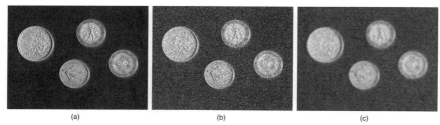

(a)   (b)   (c)

Figure 7-3. An example of image filtering. *(a)* The original image is shown. The image can be divided into features (the coins) and background. *(b)* Noise has been added to the original image, including spikes and random background fluctuations. *(c)* The image of (b) is convolved with a Gaussian PSF, showing how the convolution smoothes the image and reduces background fluctuations, although with a loss of resolution at the edges.

7.2.4.2 Rank Filters

In contrast to convolution filters, rank filters ignore some or most of the pixels in the neighborhood[23]. Because of this they have advantages for data processing, since there is no need to remove spikes or estimate empty pixels prior to application of the filter (as long as the spikes and missing pixels do not constitute a substantial portion of the background region). Rank filters are particularly useful for analysis when signal and noise are mixed together as in a microarray, because while a convolution will treat both signal and noise in the same manner, rank filters have some power to discriminate. Rank filters therefore have the advantage of potentially removing noise without affecting signal. The simplest rank filter is a median filter which looks at all pixels forming the background in a neighborhood and chooses the median value. This has the advantage not only of being computationally simple, but also of being an excellent estimate of the background. The reason for this is that the background is generally assumed to be reasonably uniform over a neighborhood-sized region, but with a few bad pixels. The key to both mean and median filters is to use a neighborhood region small enough that it has coherent variations in nonspecific hybridization which do not exceed the noise level. Recent microarrays often show considerably lower levels of nonspecific hybridization and patchiness than initial versions, making rank filters on neighborhoods good choices for background correction.

7.2.4.3 Adaptive Filters

Adaptive filters are the most complex methods of filtering. An adaptive filter uses features of the image itself to determine what type of filter to apply to an individual pixel. Uses of adaptive filters include filters which behave differently within signal areas and in background areas, allowing image enhancement based on feature recognition. Since microarrays offer very regular features (e.g. a grid of spots), adaptive filters could prove very useful in analysis. For instance, filters which automatically treat interior pixels of a spot differently from pixels at the edge, where background effects may make estimation of the exact edge difficult, are possible. Another potential use is adaptive filters that are capable of treating regions of the image with high patchiness or background differently, permitting some local background estimates and some neighborhood background estimates. Whether results of applying adaptive filters will ever justify the added computational requirements is unknown.

7.2.5 Effects of Background Correction

Figure 7-4 shows a small portion of a microarray image. This section has 25 DNA spots with intensity signals ranging from 1.8 to 168.4 (mean value of signal pixels with an average of 38.4), or from 2 to 225 (median value of signal pixels). A mean filter applied on the background pixels in the area yields a background value of 5.2. However, removal of the spikes changes this value to 3.1, even though there are only a few spikes within the image, indicating the large effect that not handling spikes correctly can have. Using the estimate with spikes, only 14 genes are considered to be significant (three times the background), while 18 genes appear significant after removing spikes. The median of the background intensity is 2, giving 19 significant genes using mean values or 18 significant genes using median values. The use of the median therefore yields results similar to the mean with the spikes removed, but with much less computation. In addition, as noted above, there are reasons to prefer median measurements, although detailed studies validating this choice for microarrays would be difficult.

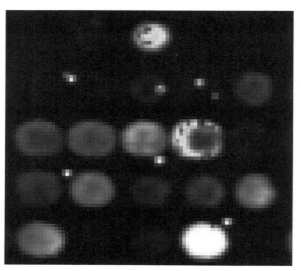

Figure 7-4. A sample image for background correction. Background correction values are generated from the image using a mean filter, a mean filter with spikes removed, and a median filter. The data is summarized in the text.

7.3 Correcting for Systematic Errors in Signals

7.3.1 Sources of Error

Once background correction has been accomplished, systematic errors within the signals generated by the fluorescent probes need to be taken into account. These systematic errors arise from a number of sources, not all of which have necessarily been identified. It must be remembered that the key feature of microarrays using probes with fluorescent dye labels is that two signals are compared, the experimental signal from probe with one color dye and the control signal from probe with a second color dye. The goal is to measure the relative copy number of mRNA between the two samples, usually reported as a ratio or log ratio between the two samples. The ratio measurement provides an inherent normalization between the two samples, so that the absolute copy number is not important, just the relative change between the experimental and control sample. This is useful since it compensates for differences in the efficiency of the reverse transcription reaction used for labeling, and also small differences between the concentrations of experimental and control mRNAs. However, for this automatic normalization by ratio to work, the intensity measurements must be on the same scale, with a concentration of the control mRNA generating the same intensity as the same concentration of experimental mRNA.

In the introduction, a number of sources of error in microarray measurements were noted. The goal of normalization will be to correct for these as completely as possible prior to data analysis.

7.3.2 Issues on Data Selection for Normalization

In order to apply a normalization procedure, control data must be selected for analysis, identifying a set of genes with a known ratio between the experimental and control conditions. Unfortunately, this is very difficult to do as knowledge of the underlying biological system in any experiment is incomplete and as stochastic processes cause natural variation even in normal cellular populations. Nevertheless, a number of choices have been proposed and these are explored below.

7.3.2.1 Housekeeping Genes

Microarrays are often viewed as a high throughput method of producing the equivalent of Northern blot data. Northern blots measure the abundance of the mRNA of an individual gene using blotting on a nitrocellulose or nylon membrane and radioactive labeling. For Northern blots, the mRNA of β-actin or another "housekeeping" gene is often used as an indicator of overall quality and amount of the isolated mRNA, so that Northerns are often demonstrated to be on the same scale by having similar amounts of β-actin. While the concept of maintaining this normalization method as one crosses from Northern analysis to microarrays is appealing, there are several problems with this approach. First, the housekeeping genes such as β-actin are highly expressed and therefore are not representative of the whole distribution of signal intensity[24]. This makes it particularly problematic to use them for normalization given the nonlinearities which occur in microarray measurements at high intensity. Second, as more microarray measurements have been made, it has become clear that there is more variation in housekeeping gene mRNA levels than initially thought, especially in situations involving disease and abnormal growth[10].

7.3.2.2 Spiked Genes

A second possible choice for normalization is the use of specific, foreign mRNAs added at known concentrations to both the control and experimental mRNAs (i.e. spiking the arrays, for example see[11]). The mRNAs are added at concentrations covering the range of concentrations present in the sample mRNAs prior to reverse transcription and labeling. Matched DNAs are spotted in multiple locations on the slide, so that the intensity of these spots provide measurements of known mRNA concentrations for normalization. This has the added advantage of providing an absolute scale of concentration for cross-slide normalization, which would permit measurements made at different times and in different laboratories to be easily compared. Unfortunately the concentrations of mRNA required for this are quite tiny, resulting in difficulties in accurately spiking the samples. For this reason, spiking is not yet widely used, though it is potentially of great value.

7.3.2.3 All Genes

A third choice for the set of normalization genes is the full complement of genes on the array. Since gene expression microarrays now routinely contain thousands or tens of thousands of genes, the likelihood that more than a couple percent of these genes will be differentially expressed in any given experiment is small. Overall, then, the gene expression levels provide their own normalization signals. Further improvement (or just peace of mind) can be made by eliminating from the gene set used for normalization all genes whose intensity ratios between the two dyes are outliers (e.g. if the average ratio prior to normalization is 0.7 ± 0.2, remove genes with ratios less than 0.1 or greater than 1.3). These genes are restored to the data set once the normalization coefficients have been determined. In practice, the removal of the few clearly differentially expressed genes from the normalization process does not seem to make a significant difference for large arrays.

7.4 Normalization Methods

Once the values (i.e. genes) to be used for normalization have been selected, the measurement type to be used and a method of correction must be chosen. Typical measurement types include the mean intensity of the signal pixels, the median intensity of the signal pixels, or the integrated intensity of the signal pixels (all with background correction). While the choice of which measurement to use is beyond the scope of this chapter, all three are routinely used by various groups. As noted above, the goal of normalization is to insure that measured intensities are proportional to mRNA concentrations. This is equivalent to modifying the intensity distributions in such a way that the ratio of experimental signal to control signal averages one and shows no intensity dependent effects for the set of normalization genes (i.e. these genes are not differentially expressed). The relationship of the experimental and control signals can be visualized by generating a scatter plot of the experimental signal intensities vs. the control signal intensities for all genes in the normalization group. Such a plot is shown for unnormalized data in Figure 7-5a. The fact that the points do not scatter about the line of slope 1 indicates that normalization is required. The signal from the experimental probe is clearly greater than that from the control probe, as the data lies significantly above the line.

7.4.1 Mean Correction

The simplest correction which can be applied to the data is a simple adjustment of the experimental or control intensities, so that the overall mean values of the two distributions are the same. This effectively scales one of the two intensity distributions to match the other. The result of this modification on the data in Figure 7-5a is shown in Figure 7-5b. As can be seen, the data now shows equal intensity overall, though the data does not lie along the line, but scatters significantly below it at high intensity. The data also lies above the line at low intensity, but this is hard to discern. Since this will automatically cause genes in the tails of the distributions (i.e. at high and low signal intensities) to appear as differentially regulated, a more complex normalization procedure is required. Also note that a curve through the points will show a clear curvature, indicative of the nonlinear effects noted above.

7.4.2 Linear Correction

The next possible correction is provided by a linear regression analysis of the data, with correction for a linear intensity dependent error. The results of such a correction applied to the data in Figure 7-5a are shown in Figure 7-5c, which shows that the data now scatters about a line of slope 1, although there is a clear nonlinearity which causes curvature at the endpoints. This curvature is likely a result of the intensity dependent quenching of signal at high intensity. The nonlinearity can be viewed as a suppression of signal in one channel at high intensity, equivalent to underestimating the mRNA copy number in either the experimental or control data. This increases the difference between points in the data at high intensity, where statistical power tends to be at a maximum. Since the effect is systematic and reproducible, the use of replicate spotting only increases the apparent statistical reliability of the measurements. The result is the creation of false positives of differential expression which appear to be significant under statistical analysis due to the high expression levels[16, 25]. The correction by linear regression analysis should not be used if nonlinearities appear in the scatter plot, and in general it is safer to use more

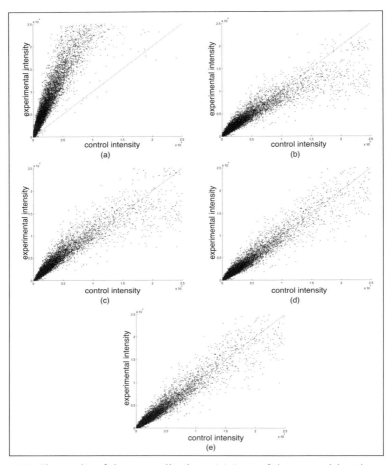

Figure 7-5. The results of data normalization. *(a)* A set of data comprising the control and experimental intensity levels from 40,000 genes is shown on a scatter plot. The plot is truncated at the top, removing a small set of genes for clarity in the image. These genes are included in the following figures. The line is a line of slope 1, which defines points corresponding to no differential regulation. *(b)* The data from (a) has been normalized by correcting for the differences in the mean level of expression. Note that the data shows clear bias at high intensity as it does not scatter about the line. *(c)* The data from (a) has been normalized using a linear regression fit. While better than the normalization shown in (b), there remains clear curvature in the data that causes points at high intensity to scatter mostly below, rather than around, the line. *(d)* The data from (a) has been normalized using a piece-wise linear fit. The data now appears linear with all data points scattering around the line. *(e)* The data from (a) has been normalized with a second order polynomial fit, which provides a correction equal or better than (d) with fewer free parameters.

advanced correction methods. It should be noted that a dye-flip experiment, where the mRNA is split into two portions, one of which has the experimental mRNA labeled with the first dye and the control mRNA labeled with the second dye, and the second of which has the dyes reversed, is quite useful for identifying these cases, although it will not eliminate the need for nonlinear correction[10].

7.4.3 Piecewise Linear Correction

The simplest nonlinear correction to apply is a piecewise linear correction, where multiple linear corrections are applied to subsections of the data. This has the advantage of being relatively easy to implement compared to a full nonlinear correction, although it does not generate a true global correction over the range of data and introduces breakpoints between regions where individual linear corrections are applied. Fortunately, given the noise levels presently observed in microarray data, the breakpoints do not appear to cause problems in most cases. The main requirement for using a piecewise linear correction is that the number of points used in any individual segment (often referred to as a bin) should be significantly larger than 1. While the size of the bin depends on the distribution of the intensities, a good rule for a modern array of thousands of genes would be at least 50 genes covering a range of intensity that appears linear. The application of a piecewise linear correction to the data of Figure 7-5a is shown in Figure 7-5d. Comparison with the linear correction of Figure 7-5c shows that the nonlinear errors at the extremes of the intensity range have been eliminated. The data now fits nicely to the expected behavior with the majority of genes not showing differential expression.

7.4.4 Curve Fitting

Although piecewise linear correction has become popular due to its ease of use and its appearance in popular software packages, a global solution provides a better method of normalization and avoids the potential for errors at interfaces between the bins created by the piecewise linear method. The danger in applying a global nonlinear correction is that complex functions could actually model the data too well, thereby allowing true differential expression to be treated as systematic error. Since second order polynomials provide adequate correction with a minimal number of parameters, they make a good choice for nonlinear, global data correction. Cubic splines have also been used, perhaps because they are included in numerous mathematical and statistical packages for curve fitting[26]. They are also a reasonably safe choice for normalization, although they do have more free parameters and thus can model the data more closely, providing a small increase in the chance that true differential expression will get normalized out. A polynomial nonlinear correction applied to the data in Figure 7-5a yields the corrected data shown in Figure 7-5e. There are no noticeable differences between this set of corrected data and that normalized with piecewise linear method (Figure 7-5d), indicating that for the typical data gathered with present methods a piecewise linear correction is adequate. However, the polynomial correction reduces significantly the number of free parameters, minimizing the possibility of introducing error.

7.5 Summary

In summary, the choice of an adequate normalization method depends on the quality of the data. The quality can generally be judged by producing a scatter plot of the experimental vs. control data. If the data shows no nonlinearities, then simple linear regression analysis can produce a normalizing curve for the data. However, it is generally the case that there is some nonlinearity due to quenching of the fluorescence of the dyes, so that nonlinear normalization is typically advisable. It is possible that technical developments will allow a return to simple adjustment by mean intensity or a linear correction, however er presently a simple nonlinear correction should be employed. Following normalization, the data is ready for statistical analysis. In general the data must be combined with replicate data from duplicate experiments and dye-flip measurements.

7.5.1 A Sample Procedure

At this point, a summary of an overall approach to data normalization for a fluorescently-labeled "two color" microarray can be given. The steps below should be used after image analysis has provided both signal and background measurements, preferably using a neighborhood method as discussed above. The outlined procedure does not provide a comprehensive method, but instead summarizes a minimal set of steps that should be taken to insure that the data can be interpreted.

1) Perform a background correction – The best choice of background correction will depend on the qualities of the image. However, for reasonably good quality images, subtracting the median value of the background pixels in the neighborhood from each signal pixel is an excellent choice.

2) Produce a scatter plot of experimental vs control intensities for all genes – Plot the background corrected experimental signal intensity against the background corrected control signal intensity together with a line of slope 1 passing through the origin. This will provide a graphical view of the data, including an indication if there is a significant chance that the gain on the scanner was set too high leading to saturation. This is identifiable by the distribution becoming horizontal or vertical as intensity increases. While the effect can be corrected for to some extent, rescanning would be advisable.

3) (OPTIONAL) Remove outliers from the gene set to be used for normalization – If desired, remove any genes from the set of genes to be used for normalization based on the point corresponding to the gene in the scatter plot of step 2 being well removed from other points. Effectively this will block genes which are likely to be significantly differentially regulated from affecting normalization.

4) Perform a piecewise linear, second order polynomial, or spline fit to the data – For the set of normalization genes, fit the appropriate curve using standard techniques, such as least squares fitting.

5) Correct all the data using the curve from the previous step – Replace any data removed in step 3. Then, for each data point, identify the corresponding point (same control intensity) on the curve calculated in step 4. Replace the experimental intensity for the gene corresponding to the data point with the corrected value (essentially the experimental intensity divided by the curve value multiplied by the control intensity).

6) Combine replicate data– Calculate the mean and standard deviation for each gene from all values which measure the same experimental to control condition (including dye-flips, replicate spots, and replicated experiments).

7) Perform analysis – Use standard statistical methods[14, 15, 27] or pattern recognition algorithms[28-36].

7.5.2 Biological Noise

In addition to the noise which arises from technical factors such as dye incorporation and fluorescence characteristics, there is "biological noise" which results from the natural variations in genetics, the stochastic nature of biological systems, and the lack of total control of experimental conditions. All of these factors can have serious implications for measurements designed to identify genes differentially regulated because of changes introduced in the experiment, since the differential expression may in reality be due to random fluctuations or other factors. An excellent example of this is given in the Rosetta compendium data, where an experiment on the yeast Saccharomyces cerevisiae was repeated as precisely as possible 63 times[13]. There remained substantial variations in the level of gene expression measured on the microarrays. The variation was completely gene dependent, with some genes varying substantially throughout the control experiments, while others showed only small variations consistent with noise arising from technological factors.

The presence of these natural variations even in a very controlled experiment stresses the importance of performing repeated experiments. It should be remembered that although microarray experiments provide a relatively inexpensive way to measure the gene expression of thousands of genes, followup by more laborious and costly measurements are generally still required. It is therefore logical to repeat the inexpensive experiment to verify a tentative result prior to embarking on more costly measurements. In addition, most new methods of determining differential expression rely on repeated measurements to determine a confidence measure[14, 16, 27]. This is a far more reliable and powerful method than merely listing genes which undergo two- or three-fold changes. In the case of experiments performed with the goal of performing pattern recognition, the repeated experiments provide a rudimentary measure of uncertainty for each expression level, which can be useful for advanced data analysis methods[36].

7.6 Conclusion

Gene expression microarrays provide a powerful tool for probing the inner workings of cells under a variety of conditions. The opportunity to perform genome-wide measurements of gene expression may provide insights into unforeseen mechanisms underlying cellular development, disease, and growth. However, as with any technology, proper data handling is essential to maximize the usefulness of the gathered data and to interpret the resulting deluge of numbers. Since the complexity of the data being generated by functional genomics is expected to dwarf that of the genomic data sets[37], it is essential that the data be handled properly to avoid misinterpretation. Part of that careful handling is proper background correction and data normalization, to take into account hybridization effects such as nonspecific binding, dye incorporation effects tied to specific sequences, differences in intensity responses of the dyes to laser excitation, and quenching effects of the dyes at high intensities. While these effects can be corrected by normalization, there are additional effects which present greater difficulties. One problem is that it appears that certain specific mRNA sequences cannot be easily converted to labeled cDNA with both possible dyes. The result is that certain sequences will have their signal suppressed in either the control or experimental data, resulting in false estimates of up- or down-regulation[10]. This is one reason for the use of dye-flips in an analysis.

Background correction and data normalization provide a method to make the results of a single microarray measurement meaningful. However, they do not address other issues of equal importance, such as the reliability of a given measurement and the presence of biological noise. These issues can only be addressed by replicating the experimental protocol where possible, and sampling a population where appropriate (as in a study involving human responses to chemotherapy or other cases where replication is impossible). The replication also permits more useful data analysis, permitting the generation of significance values in statistical measurements or providing uncertainty estimates to the measurements for pattern recognition algorithms. As such, replication in a microarray study should be taken as a fundamental step in experimental design[38].

As microarray technology matures, the precision of the measurements made will improve, allowing ever more accurate views into the transcriptional life of cells under a variety of conditions. However, data cleaning will also be needed to maximize the usefulness of the measurements. The type of corrections applied will change with time and technology, however the standard scientific rules; replication of experiments, careful experimental design, and an understanding of the systems used; cannot be broken without the risk of misinterpretation. Such misinterpretation can be costly, leading to pointless experiments aimed at confirming nonexistent effects. By keeping in mind the system used to perform a measurement, by modeling the errors and correcting for them as best as possible, and by careful interpretation of results, the maximum information will always be retrievable.

Acknowledgements

We would like to thank Dr. Burton Eisenberg and Dr. Andrew Godwin of the Fox Chase Cancer Center for providing microarray data for analysis. We would also like to thank Dr. Yuesheng Li, Director of the Microarray Facility at Fox Chase, for assistance. This work was supported by the NIH Comprehensive Cancer Center Core Grant CA06927 to Dr. R. Young, by the NIH Ovarian SPORE P50 CA83638 grant to Dr. R. Ozols, and by the Pew Foundation.

References

1. **Ramdas L, Coombes KR, Baggerly K, Abruzzo L, Highsmith WE, Krogmann T, Hamilton SR, Zhang W**: Sources of nonlinearity in cDNA microarray expression measurements. *Genome Biol 2001*; 2.

2. **Stears RL, Getts RC, Gullans SR**: A novel, sensitive detection system for high-density microarrays using dendrimer technology. *Physiol Genomics 2000*; 3:93-9.

3. **Cavalieri D, Townsend JP, Hartl DL**: Manifold anomalies in gene expression in a vineyard isolate of Saccharomyces cerevisiae revealed by DNA microarray analysis. *Proc Natl Acad Sci U S A 2000*; 97:12369-74.

4. **Coller HA, Grandori C, Tamayo P, Colbert T, Lander ES, Eisenman RN, Golub TR**: Expression analysis with oligonucleotide microarrays reveals that MYC regulates genes involved in growth, cell cycle, signaling, and adhesion. *Proc Natl Acad Sci U S A 2000*; 97:3260-5.

5. **Maxwell SA, Davis GE**: Differential gene expression in p53-mediated apoptosis-resistant vs. apoptosis-sensitive tumor cell lines. *Proc Natl Acad Sci U S A 2000*; 97:13009-14.

6. **Cho RJ, Campbell MJ, Winzeler EA, Steinmetz L, Conway A, Wodicka L, Wolfsberg TG, Gabrielian AE, Landsman D, Lockhart DJ, Davis RW**: A genome-wide transcriptional analysis of the mitotic cell cycle. *Mol Cell 1998*; 2:65-73.

7. **Chu S, DeRisi J, Eisen M, Mulholland J, Botstein D, Brown PO, Herskowitz I**: The transcriptional program of sporulation in budding yeast. *Science 1998*; 282:699-705.

8. **Iyer VR, Eisen MB, Ross DT, Schuler G, Moore T, Lee JCF, Trent JM, Staudt LM, Hudson J, Jr., Boguski MS, Lashkari D, Shalon D, Botstein D, Brown PO**: The transcriptional program in the response of human fibroblasts to serum. *Science 1999*; 283:83-7.

9. **Spellman PT, Sherlock G, Zhang MQ, Iyer VR, Anders K, Eisen MB, Brown PO, Botstein D, Futcher B**: Comprehensive identification of cell cycle-regulated genes of the yeast Saccharomyces cerevisiae by microarray hybridization. *Mol Biol Cell 1998*; 9:3273-97.

10. **Tseng GC, Oh MK, Rohlin L, Liao JC, Wong WH**: Issues in cDNA microarray analysis: quality filtering, channel normalization, models of variations and assessment of gene effects. *Nucleic Acids Res 2001*; 29:2549-57.

11. **Schuchhardt J, Beule D, Malik A, Wolski E, Eickhoff H, Lehrach H, Herzel H**: Normalization strategies for cDNA microarrays. *Nucleic Acids Research 2000*; 28:e47.

12. **Hughes TR, Mao M, Jones AR, Burchard J, Marton MJ, Shannon KW, Lefkowitz SM, Ziman M, Schelter JM, Meyer MR, Kobayashi S, Davis C, Dai H, He YD, Stephaniants SB, Cavet G, Walker WL, West A, Coffey E, Shoemaker DD, Stoughton R, Blanchard AP, Friend SH, Linsley PS**: Expression profiling using microarrays fabricated by an ink-jet oligonucleotide synthesizer. *Nat Biotechnol 2001*; 19:342-7.

13. *Hughes TR, Marton MJ, Jones AR, Roberts CJ, Stoughton R, Armour CD, Bennett HA, Coffey E, Dai H, He YD, Kidd MJ, King AM, Meyer MR, Slade D, Lum PY, Stepaniants SB, Shoemaker DD, Gachotte D, Chakraburtty K, Simon J, Bard M, Friend SH*: Functional discovery via a compendium of expression profiles. *Cell 2000*; 102:109-26.

14. *Ideker T, Thorsson V, Siegel AF, Hood LE*: Testing for differentially-expressed genes by maximum-likelihood analysis of microarray data. *J Comput Biol 2000*; 7:805-17.

15. *Kerr MK, Afshari CA, Bennett L, Bushel P, Martinez J, Walker NJ, Churchill GA*: Statistical analysis of a gene expression microarray experiment with replication. *Statistica Sinica 2001*.

16. *Kerr MK, Martin M, Churchill GA*: Analysis of variance for gene expression microarray data. *J Comput Biol 2000*; 7:819-37.

17. *Brown CS, Goodwin PC, Sorger PK*: Image metrics in the statistical analysis of DNA microarray data. *Proc Natl Acad Sci U S A 2001*; 98:8944-9.

18. *Jähne B*: Practical handbook on image processing for scientific applications. Boca Raton, Fla., *CRC Press*, 1997.

19. *Russ JC*: The image processing handbook. Boca Raton, FL, *CRC Press*, 1999.

20. *Huang Q, Dom B, Megiddo N, Niblack W*: Segmenting and representing background in color images. *Proc 1996 Intern Conf on Patt Recog 1996*:13 - 17.

21. *Hegde P, Qi R, Abernathy K, Gay C, Dharap S, Gaspard R, Hughes JE, Snesrud E, Lee N, Quackenbush J*: A concise guide to cDNA microarray analysis. *Biotechniques 2000*; 29:548-50, 552-4, 556 passim.

22. *Wang X, Ghosh S, Guo SW*: Quantitative quality control in microarray image processing and data acquisition. *Nucleic Acids Res 2001*; 29:E75-5.

23. *Chen Y, Dougherty ER, Bittner ML*: Ratio-based decisions and the quantitative analysis of cDNA microarray images. *J. of Biomedical Optics* 1997; 2:364-374.

24. *Yang YH, Dudoit S, Luu P, Speed TP*: Normalization for cDNA microarray data. Berkeley, *University of California at Berkeley,Technical Report* 578, 2000.

25. *Claverie JM*: Computational methods for the identification of differential and coordinated gene expression. *Hum Mol Genet 1999*; 8:1821-32.

26. *Press WH*: Numerical recipes in C : the art of scientific computing. Cambridge [Cambridgeshire] ; New York, *Cambridge University Press*, 1997.

27. *Newton MA, Kendziorski CM, Richmond CS, Blattner FR, Tsui KW*: On differential variability of expression ratios: improving statistical inference about gene expression changes from microarray data. *J Comput Biol 2001*; 8:37-52.

28. *Alizadeh AA, Eisen MB, Davis RE, Ma C, Lossos IS, Rosenwald A, Boldrick JC, Sabet H, Tran T, Yu X, Powell JI, Yang L, Marti GE, Moore T, Hudson J, Jr., Lu L, Lewis DB, Tibshirani R, Sherlock G, Chan WC, Greiner TC, Weisenburger DD, Armitage JO, Warnke R, Staudt LM, et al.*: Distinct types of diffuse large B-cell lymphoma identified by gene expression profiling. *Nature 2000*; 403:503-11.

29. *Bittner M, Meltzer P, Chen Y, Jiang Y, Seftor E, Hendrix M, Radmacher M, Simon R, Yakhini Z, Ben-Dor A, Sampas N, Dougherty E, Wang E, Marincola F, Gooden C, Lueders J, Glatfelter A, Pollock P, Carpten J, Gillanders E, Leja D, Dietrich K, Beaudry C, Berens M, Alberts D, Sondak V*: Molecular classification of cutaneous malignant melanoma by gene expression profiling. *Nature 2000*; 406:536-40.

30. *Brown MP, Grundy WN, Lin D, Cristianini N, Sugnet CW, Furey TS, Ares M, Jr., Haussler D*: Knowledge-based analysis of microarray gene expression data by using support vector machines. *Proc Natl Acad Sci U S A 2000*; 97:262-7.

31. *Eisen MB, Spellman PT, Brown PO, Botstein D*: Cluster analysis and display of genome-wide expression patterns. *Proc Natl Acad Sci U S A 1998*; 95:14863-8.

32. *Heyer LJ, Kruglyak S, Yooseph S*: Exploring expression data: identification and analysis of coexpressed genes. *Genome Res 1999*; 9:1106-15.

33. *Lukashin AV, Fuchs R*: Analysis of temporal gene expression profiles: clustering by simulated annealing and determining the optimal number of clusters. *Bioinformatics 2001*; 17:405-14.

34. *Tamayo P, Slonim D, Mesirov J, Zhu Q, Kitareewan S, Dmitrovsky E, Lander ES, Golub TR*: Interpreting patterns of gene expression with self-organizing maps: methods and application to hematopoietic differentiation. *Proc Natl Acad Sci U S A 1999*; 96:2907-12.

35. *Bidaut G, Moloshok TD, Grant JD, Manion FJ, Ochs MF*: Bayesian Decomposition analysis of gene expression in yeast deletion mutants; in Johnson K, Lin S (eds): Methods of Microarray Data Analysis II. Boston, *Kluwer Academic*, 2002, pp.105-122.

36. *Moloshok TD, Klevecz RR, Grant JD, Manion FJ, Speier WI, Ochs MF*: Application of Bayesian Decomposition for analysing microarray data. *Bioinformatics 2002*; 18:566-575.

37. *Bittner M, Meltzer P, Trent J*: Data analysis and integration: of steps and arrows. *Nat Genet 1999*; 22:213-5.

38. *Kerr MK, Churchill GA*: Statistical design and the analysis of gene expression microarray data. *Genet Res 2001*; 77:123-8.

QUANTITATIVE COMPARISON OF IMAGE ANALYSIS SOFTWARE

Diane Moody, Bassem Fadlia, Abhay Singh, Swapnal Shah, Lauren McIntyre
Genomics Database Facility, Purdue University

Contact:
Lauren McIntyre, Ph.D.
1150 Lilly Hall, Purdue University, West Lafayette, IN 47907 U.S.A.
E-mail: lmcintyre@purdue.edu

0-9664027-5-8/02/$0.00+$.50   *From:* **Microarray Image Analysis-Nuts & Bolts** (pp.155-166)
©2002 by DNA Press, LLC   Edited by: S. Shah and G. Kamberova

8.1 Introduction

An important, and often overlooked, step in microarray experimentation is the acquisition of quantitative data that represent the level of gene expression for each element on the array. This step is typically accomplished using a software package to identify individual elements from a digital image of an array, and quantifying the amount of signal within a defined region representing each array element. As genomic efforts scale up and technology becomes more affordable, 'automated' image quantification is a desirable software feature. Several software packages are available to accomplish this task, and each software package has its own features tailored for ease of use and specific applications. When choosing software to process a large number of images, three important criteria include: 1) user interface and throughput that can be achieved when processing multiple images, 2) the reliability with which quantitative gene expression data can be extracted from the image, and 3) the accuracy with which the data reflect signals from the array. Reliability of data acquisition is important because it impacts the power, or the chance of finding a significant difference, of the experiment[1]. In other words, variation introduced during the data acquisition process may inhibit the detection of true differences in gene expression among experimental treatments. In order to compensate for this reduced power, additional replication is needed. When additional replication is not feasible, it becomes critical that each step of the experimental process is evaluated in order to maximize reliability of the data generated. Thus, it is important that the reliability of the acquisition of quantitative data from array images is considered. It is also essential that the quantitation of microarray data accurately reflect the hybridization signal of each array element. Although it is difficult to determine what the actual expression value should be, multiple analysis using different programs can be helpful in identifying systematic problems. A final consideration in microarray data acquisition is the amount of time and user input required to analyze multiple images. In some situations, it may be possible to manually identify microarray elements, while other situations may require automated processing to avoid a bottleneck in the microarray experimentation process. Ease of use, flexibility, and other specific options of software packages may also be important considerations for specific applications.

In this chapter, we describe a systematic evaluation of three microarray data acquisition software packages. In order to provide a benchmark to which investigators may compare the reliability of data acquisition in their own experiments, we have evaluated these software packages using a variety of different types of arrays (macro and microarrays; glass and nylon; cDNA and bacterial). The three software packages considered include: ImageQuant (Amersham Biosciences-http://www.apbiotech.com), QuantArray (Packard

Bioscience/PerkinElmer Life Sciences - http://www.packardbioscience.com), and ImaGene (BioDiscovery - http://www.biodiscovery.com). The reliability, accuracy, and throughput of data generated from each type of microarray and each software package are discussed.

8.2 Comparison of Data Acquisition Software

8.2.1 Experimental Design

Eight images representing different types of microarray formats of varying complexity were selected (Figure 8-1). The images are numbered 1 through 8 according to their complexity. For example, image 1 is a macroarray of 1,536 bacterial colonies arranged in a single grid, and image 7 is a glass slide cDNA microarray including 15,360 elements arranged in 3 large blocks with several subgrids inside each block (.tiff files of images are accessible through our web site, www.genomics.purdue.edu/services/testimage.html). These images provide a set of common test images that may be used to evaluate additional software packages. Where possible, data were acquired from each image three times using each software package.

8.2.2 Data Acquisition

A different user acquired the data from each software package. Users of ImageQuant and ImaGene were new to the software, while the QuantArray data were obtained by a user familiar with the program. ImaGene data were obtained using the spot-finding feature with minimal manual adjustment of individual spots. QuantArray data were also obtained using the spot-finding feature, but considerable manual manipulation was done to generate the data used in this evaluation. Results are presented for ImageQuant data generated using the volume option. Analyses were also done using data generated using the maximum integer and median options, and similar results were obtained (data not shown). We also wanted to evaluate a fully automated system. We tested the batch feature of the ImaGene software as follows. We selected the two simplest images (1 and 2) and saved each image three times. We used the grid developed from image one and batch processed the six remaining images. We then used the batch mode to generate data for images 4, 5, 6 and 7.

8.2.3 Statistical Analysis

Reliability of data acquisition was evaluated in three ways: a Pearson correlation coefficient, the kappa statistic, and Bowker's test for Symmetry (Figure 8-1). Analyses were performed using the 'proc corr' and 'proc freq' commands of the SAS statistical analysis package [2]. High Pearson correlations (~1) and

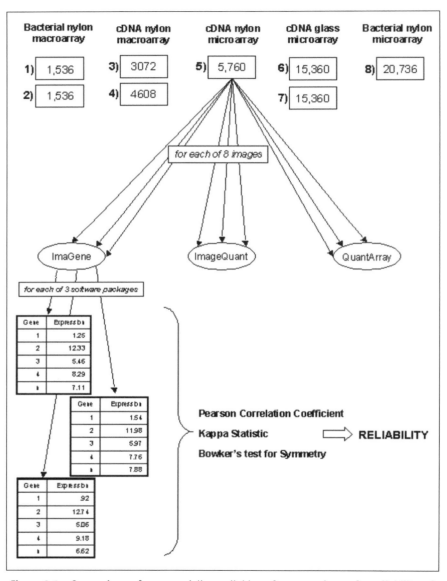

Figure 8-1: Comparison of commercially available software packages for reliability of data acquisition.

Figure 8-1: Comparison of commercially available software packages for reliability of data acquisition. Eight array images representing different solid support materials (glass versus nylon), densities (microarray versus macroarray; total number of elements on each array is shown [#]), and types of arrays (cDNA versus bacterial) were used. Each image was analyzed three times using three different software packages:

ImageQuant (Amersham Biosciences - http://www.apbiotech.com),
QuantArray (Packard Bioscience/PerkinElmer Life Sciences - http://www.packardbio-science.com), and
Imagene (BioDiscovery - http://www.biodiscovery.com) generating three complete data sets from each of the three software packages where possible.

Image numbers 1 through 8 correspond to the .tiff files found at www.genomics.pur-due.edu/database/array/images.html.

kappa statistics, and non-significant Bowker's tests are desirable in that they indicate the software reliably identified and quantified microarray elements (i.e. similar results were generated each time the images were analyzed). For each microarray and each software package, Pearson correlation coefficients were calculated between pairs of data. The average of the three correlation coefficients were calculated to represent the repeatability of the data generated using each software package. As these correlations may overestimate concordance when data are not normally distributed (i.e. when there are a large number genes with low hybridization signals) the data were also examined categorically. For this analysis, each spot was categorized into one of four levels (Q1, Q2, Q3, or Q4) based on its relative expression (Q1=lowest quartile of expression; Q2=2nd quartile of expression; Q3=3rd quartile of expression; Q4=highest quartile of expression). A frequency table of the quartiles from two independent analyses of each image is computed (e.g Table 8-1). The Kappa coefficient is estimated and Bowker's test for symmetry is then performed using the frequency tables. The Kappa coefficient is the chance corrected measure of agreement, and indicates the likelihood that expression levels will fall into the same categories, or quartiles, when the data acquisition process is repeated. This measure takes into account unequal marginal distributions and can be interpreted in the same way as a correlation coefficient[1]. Bowker's test for symmetry tests the null hypothesis that discrepancies, or genes with expression levels falling into different quartiles in different analyses, are evenly distributed in the upper and lower portions of the frequency table. Rejection of this null hypothesis using Bowker's test indicates a systematic difference in data acquired from two analyses of the same image.

The accuracy with which each software package identifies and quantitates each array element is difficult to calculate because the true expression level of each element is not known. We have calculated the Spearman correlation coefficients between the average expression values generated by different software packages in order to provide a general comparison among the packages. The Spearman correlation is calculated based on the relative ranking of the expression values generated by each software package, and was used because expression values from different packages did not display the same mean or range. Thus, a high Spearman correlation coefficient (close to 1) indicates the relative ranking of array elements was similar between software packages.

8.3 Results

8.3.1 Interface and Throughput

The relative ease of use of different software packages will depend upon the personal preferences and experience of each user. However, some significant differences in the capabilities of the three software packages evaluated were noted. The ImaGene software was the only package that identified elements from all of the arrays, including a complex nylon microarray of bacterial colonies (image 8). ImaGene software was flexible and easily adjustable to accommodate different array layouts. Quantarray successfully generated data from all images except image 8. This package was also flexible and adaptable to multiple layouts, although it was not able to handle the large, complex image 8. The QuantArray software also seemed to require more manual intervention to correctly identify spots, while the automatic spot-finding feature of ImaGene was generally successful. ImageQuant was somewhat limited in its applications because it could only accommodate images where all spots were equidistant from one another. Because of this limitation, ImageQuant successfully generated data only from images 1, 2, 6, and 7, but not from the remaining four arrays in our evaluation. The automated batch feature of the ImaGene package was easy to use and time efficient

8.3.2 Reliability

The average Pearson correlation coefficients were greater than .95 for most analyses (Table 8-1). Exceptions include data from images 8 (Pearson= 0.872), and 4 (Pearson=0.91) using ImaGene software. Image 8 is a complex bacterial array with over 20,000 array elements, and ImaGene was the only package that successfully generated data from this image. It is not surprising that the reliability of data from this image is lowest, although values greater than 0.8 are generally considered excellent[1]. The reduced average Pearson correlation coefficient for image 4 results from low correlations with one data set; the correlation between the other two datasets was 1.0. Thus, the average correlation for this image may reflect user error in capturing a single data set.

Table 8-1: Average Pearson Correlation Coefficients. Pearson correlation coefficients were calculated for pairs of data. The average of three is shown to represent the reliability of each software package when analyzing the same image multiple times.

Image Number	Type of Array[a]	Number of Array Elements	Average Pearson Correlation Coefficient		
			ImaGene	QuantArray	ImageQuant
1	Nylon bacterial	1,536	0.998	0.999	0.990
2	Nylon bacterial	1,536	0.993	0.995	0.993
3	Nylon cDNA	3,072	0.999	NA[b]	NA
4	Nylon cDNA	4,608	0.913	0.974	NA
5	Nylon cDNA	5,760	0.995	0.960	NA
6	Glass cDNA (Cy3)	15,360	0.998	1.0	0.971
7	Glass cDNA (Cy5)	15,360	0.998	1.0	0.960
8	Nylon bacterial	20,736	0.872	NA	NA

a For a description of the images analyzed, see Figure 1 and:
http://www.genomics.purdue.edu/services/testimage.html
b NA: The software package was unsuccessful in identifying and quantitating data for these images.

An example of a frequency table used to calculate the Kappa coefficients is provided in Table 8-2. Average Kappa coefficients were high (Table 8-3), but slightly lower than the Pearson correlation coefficients, as expected. Significant differences in symmetry were found for three images. Two of those images (4 and 8) have been discussed above. The asymmetry detected for image 5 may reflect a systematic difference in manual adjustment of individual spots, as no evidence of asymmetry was found in the data generated for this image by QuantArray. This result indicates that some array layouts may require more supervision and adjustment of the automatic spot-finding feature than what was given to the ImaGene analysis in our evaluation.

8.3.3 Accuracy

Spearman correlation coefficients indicate data acquired from ImaGene and QuantArray are very similar, while no significant correlation was seen between these data and data generated by ImageQuant (Table 8-4, Figures 8-2 and 8-3). The reason for the extreme difference in the ImageQuant data may be due to the different use of the grid to capture information. This difference illustrates that variation among data acquisition software packages does exist and needs to be carefully examined during software selection. We do not know the true expression levels of the genes represented on these arrays, so it is impossible to say with certainty which data most accurately reflect the true gene expression levels. However, the high correlation between the ImaGene and QuantArray data is noteworthy.

The performance of the batch feature of the ImaGene software is also reflected in Table 8-4. The correlation of the ImaGene batch data to the QuantArray data is very similar to the correlation between the original Imagene and QuantArray data for images 1 and 2 (Spearman correlation coefficients = 0.944 and 0.931, respectively.) However, the correlations for the batch data of the more complex images 5, 6, and 7 were much lower (Spearman correlation coefficients less than 0.75). This result indicates that the current batch feature works well for simple images but may require additional adjustment when used with complex or multi-grid arrays.

Table 8-2: Frequency table. An example of a frequency table generated from two analyses of a glass cDNA microarray using ImaGene software. Numbers on the diagonal represent array elements that fell within the same quartile of expression in both analyses. Numbers above and below the diagonal represent array elements that fell into different quartiles of expression in the two analyses. The Kappa coeffiecient was 0.9961 and Bowker's test for symmetry failed to reject the null that the table was symmetric (p=0.94).

Quartiles of Expression: 2nd Analysis	Quartiles of Expression: 1st Analysis			
	Q1	Q2	Q3	Q4
Q1	3825	8	2	5
Q2	8	3827	4	1
Q3	4	3	3829	4
Q4	3	2	5	3830

Table 8-3: Average Kappa Statistics and Results from Bowker's Test for Symmetry. Kappa statistics were calculated for each pair of data after categorizing based on quartile of expression. The average of three Kappa statistics is shown to represent the reliability of each software package when analyzing the same image multiple times. Bowker's test for symmetry was used to test for a systematic change in expression values between analysis.

Image Number	Type of Array[a]	Number of Array Elements	Average Kappa Statistic ImaGene	QuantArray	ImageQuant
1	Nylon bacterial	1,536	0.978	0.977	0.944
2	Nylon bacterial	1,536	0.949	0.949	0.931
3	Nylon cDNA	3,072	0.977	NA[b]	NA
4	Nylon cDNA	4,608	0.706[c]	0.848	NA
5	Nylon cDNA	5,760	0.837[c]	0.906	NA
6	Glass cDNA (Cy3)	15,360	0.997	1.0	0.929
7	Glass cDNA (Cy5)	15,360	0.996	1.0	0.943
8	Nylon bacterial	20,736	0.786[c]	NA	NA

a For a description of the images analyzed, see Figure 1 and http://www.genomics.purdue.edu/services/testimage.html

b NA: The software package was unsuccessful in identifying and quantitating data for these images.

c At least one of three Bowker's tests for symmetry was significant (p<.05)

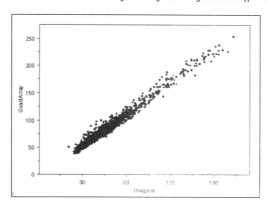

Figure 8-2: Relative expression levels generated by ImaGene and QuantArray software packages. The average relative expression levels generated for a bacterial nylon macroarray with 1,536 elements is compared for ImaGene (x axis) and QuantArray (y axis) software packages.

Table 8-4: Spearman Correlation Coefficients. The relative ranking of average expression levels was compared between software packages by calculating the Spearman Correlation Coefficient.

Image Number	Type of Array[a]	Number of Array Elements	Spearman Correlation Coefficient			
			ImageQuant/ QuantArray	ImageQuant/ ImaGene	ImaGene/ QuantArray	ImaGene[b]/ QuantArray
1	Nylon bacterial	1,536	-0.01	-0.010	.9870	.986
2	Nylon bacterial	1,536	-0.012	-0.002	0.991	0.984
3	Nylon cDNA	3,072	NA[c]	NA	NA	NA
4	Nylon cDNA	4,608	NA	NA	0.898	0.911
5	Nylon cDNA	5,760	NA	NA	0.711	0.702
6	Glass cDNA(Cy3)	15,360	0.178	0.171	0.943	0.982
7	Glass cDNA(Cy5)	15,360	0.187	0.176	0.930	0.861
8	Nylon bacterial	20,736	NA	NA	NA	NA

a For a complete description of the images analyzed, see: www.genomics.purdue.edu/database/array/images.html
b Images were analyzed using the batch processing feature of the ImaGene software.
c NA: One or both of the software packages was unsuccessful in identifying and quantitating data for these images.

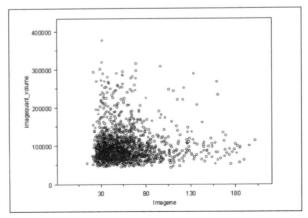

Figure 8-3a: Relative expression levels generated by ImaGene and ImageQuant software packages. The average relative expression levels generated for a bacterial nylon macroarray with 1,536 elements is compared for ImaGene (x axis) and ImageQuant (y axis) software packages. ImageQuant plot is using the volume option.

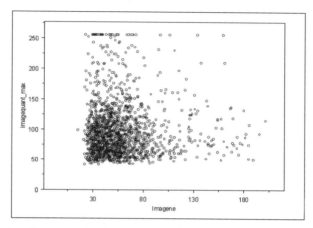

Figure 8-3b: Relative expression levels generated by ImaGene and ImageQuant software packages. The average relative expression levels generated for a bacterial nylon macroarray with 1,536 elements is compared for ImaGene (x axis) and ImageQuant (y axis) software packages. ImageQuant plot is using the maximum integer option

8.4 Conclusions

In summary we find that ImageQuant is not comparable to QuantArray and ImaGene software, and that ImageQuant has difficulty with larger and more complex arrays. The results presented are for the volume option. We also examined the maximum integer option (Figure 3b) and found that a ceiling value exists for this option. In the simple images (1 and 2), a noticeable number of the spots were at the ceiling value, and for images 6 and 7 approximately half the spots were at the ceiling value. For this reason we would discourage use of this option. The correlation between ImaGene and QuantArray was not improved by the use of the maximum integer or median options. This indicates that the grid itself is not comparable to the spot finding algorithms of Imagene and QuantArray. ImaGene and QuantArray generate similar results with good reliability. An investigator's choice between them will depend primarily on the type of images needing quantification, and the subjective interaction of the investigator with the software interface. QuantArray was not able to analyze two of the multi-grid nylon test images, while ImaGene was able to quantify all images. ImaGene batch mode worked well for the simpler images but not as well for the more complex images, pointing to areas of possible improvement for both vendors.

Acknowledgements

The authors would like to thank Drs. Chris Bidwell, Clint Chapple, Avtar Handa, Lou Sherman, and Ms. Jo Cusumano and Ms. Tatsiana Datsenka for providing images and/or data for this review. This work was funded through the Purdue Agricultural Research Station, a USDA-IFAFS grant N0014-94-1-0318 (LM), and the Purdue University Academic Reinvestment Program (LMM, WA, DM).

References

1. *Fleiss, J:* Statistical Methods for Rates and Proportions. Wiley and Sons, New York, NY, 1981.

2. *SAS*. Version 8. The SAS Institute, Cary, NC, 1999.

CHAPTER

DNA ARRAY INFORMATION WORKFLOW AND DATA MANAGEMENT

Manuel Duval, Ph.D.

Contact:
Manuel Duval

Pfizer Global Research Development,
Fresnes Laboratories, 3-9 rue de la loge, 94265 Fresnes, France
E-mail: manuel.duval@pfizer.com

0-9664027-5-8/02/$0.00+$.50   *From:* **Microarray Image Analysis-Nuts & Bolts** (pp.167-184)
©2002 by DNA Press, LLC   Edited by: S. Shah and G. Kamberova

9.1 Genomics Data Types: Gene Sequence and Expression Data

9.1.1 Sequence Data Set

A gene has two informational contents: the code for the protein it speci-fies and the regulatory elements which determine when, where and how much of this protein is produced. Both attributes are written in DNA sequences. Genomics is aiming to describe the mechanisms that govern a biological system at the genome level. Therefore, the prerequisite is to gather both characteris-tics of as many genes that compose a given organism. The very first step is to collect whole genome sequences for biologically relevant model organisms[1, 17]. The next step is to build an inventory of all genes that build the model organ-isms[5, 19, 30]. This is an on going task that is making use of available cDNA sequences, gene prediction algorithms and genome comparison (e.g. Human vs Mouse)[13, 22]. The completion of the catalogue of the whole gene set has already been done for yeast[14]. For higher organisms, elements of complexity present a greater challenge in attempting to reach the same goal : among them, the repetitive elements, the increase in size of the introns, the experimental problem to approach chromosomes telomeric and centromeric regions for sequencing and more significantly, splice variation. Alternative splicing means that the relationship between a gene and the mRNA template it specifies is not simply a one-to-one but in most cases a one-to-many. Splice variation has an impact on how genes are listed and how expression data are assigned to them. Nevertheless, there are no major technical obstacles that prevent the obtain-ment of all gene and transcript sequence data. It is just a matter of time before genomics will take advantage of a comprehensive list of gene sequences for a series of higher organisms. DNA sequences are linear strings of data, and there-fore require relatively little ancillary information. This first set of data repre-sents the foundation from which the second type of data have to be captured: expression data.

9.1.2 Gene Expression Data Set

Regulatory elements that drive gene expression are short sequences dis-tributed across long DNA segments around the exons[21]. These elements act in combination to specify expression pattern and are turned on or off depending on the presence of trans-acting factors. Therefore, there is currently no way (at least for eukaryotic organisms) to predict the expression pattern of genes by uniquely examining the genome sequences. Consequently this information has to be collected by experimental measurements of gene expression. Numerous methods are available for detecting and quantifying gene expression levels; Northern blots, S1 nuclease protection[29], differential display[8], sequencing of cDNA libraries (EST program)[10], serial analysis of gene expression[11], real time

PCR[25] and the Lynx's MPPS technology [4]. The more versatile and flexible high throughput methods are gridded cDNA and oligonucleotide microarrays[7, 24, 31] available in various forms, ranging from spotted nylon filters[26] to glass based arrays[9] and photolithographic microchips manufactured by Affymetrix[20]. DNA arrays' technologies provide the means to get gene expression data at the genome scale. It allows one to obtain spatial and temporal information about gene expression (e.g. in which tissue the gene is expressed) and dynamic information (to which extent the expression pattern of one given gene relates to those of others). Microarrays serve the objective of assigning expression data to gene sequence data. Ultimately, all coding sequences will be assigned an expression pattern. All together these two data sets will be used to construct models to describe organisms. Yet, gene expression data is not only a number. DNA arrays deliver relative occurrence values. Depending on the normalization protocol applied to treat the DNA array raw data output, the final outcome is a reference either to the total amount of mRNAs or a relative amount between two different tissues or two different time points

9.2 Data Management

Expression data is associated with a series of attributes. Among them are the experimental design, the array design, the sample preparation, the hybridization procedures and parameters and the normalization strategy. Therefore, readouts from DNA microarrays only make sense in the light of a suite of supporting information defining the type of chip used, the nature of the tissue samples involved, which kind of controls were used (e.g. spike controls), and so on. Keeping always in mind that expression data have to be pointed back to a gene or to a sequence it refers to, data management is required at three different levels: first, central to the manufacture of DNA arrays there is a need for a management system capable of tracking samples through every phase of processing, from initial sample receipt to data capture[12]. This information system has to ensure the integrity of the data by keeping track of the identity of the clone through the complex laboratory process. Secondly, within one research unit, data collected and analysis generated during the course of the process must be stored and preserved in a way that make them readily available for statistical and biological analysis[16]. Inherently, such system has to be able to at least comply to the following requirements: (i) accommodate large quantities of data set; (ii) able to hold all associated information; (iii) able to handle multiple projects simultaneously; (iv) allow platform-independent browsing of the output. Finally comes the issue of the portability of the data across different research laboratories and more ambitiously across different gene expression data acquisition platforms in addition to DNA microarray. Such a task raises the need for standardization of both gene expression outcome and accessory information. Significant efforts of the genomics community are put into the definition of common standards for the description of DNA array experiments[2, 6]. This lead to the concept of a minimum set of attributes that needs to accompany any gene expression data in order to ensure its interpretability and exchangeability. These efforts contributed to the definition of a gene expression data structure and the development a data exchange format based on XML.

The starting point for the production of DNA arrays is to have access to a collection of DNA reagents that will ultimately be assayed with complex probes. At this point, two options are available.

Several providers (Apogent Technologies, Clontech, Stratagene, R&D Systems, Research Genetics/Invitrogen, Mergen, and others) supply ready-to-use DNA arrays. Spread sheet files come with them that give the position of clones with respect to their identifier. Depending on which image acquisition platform is used, these files can be directly read by the data acquisition software. The GenePix Pro software which runs the GenePix 4000 scanners (Axon Instrument) reads a tab delimited text file which links the physical location of the spot with their ID. GenePix converts this file into a GAL file (which stands for Gene Array List) which is used to assign scanning outcome data to each spot ID. The output file is also a tab delimited text file with a header containing useful information on how data acquisition was performed, among them the pixel size, the PMT value and the laser power. It also incorporates barcode information provided the slide is featuring it.

9.3 Data Management Tools

In house oligonucleotide or cDNA arrays production is a second option for high throughput expression profiling: whether the DNA reagents come from a cDNA library or a set of oligonucleotides, both approaches require the same downstream system to design the array. Immobilized DNA featured on the slide is referred to as target. Targets DNA are physically accommodated into microtiter plates. This represents both the storage format and the holder with which DNA is presented to be automatically arrayed. Because the DNA targets represent the primary resource, it is often desirable to make back-up of the plates and to always keep a master plate from which the original clones can be retrieved. This holds true particularly for cDNA libraries which represent the outcome of a complex EST program and clone selection.

Therefore, it makes sense to implement a database aimed at holding information about source plates such as plate number, date of production or shipping, clone ID in each plate and how many times the plate has been used and thawed. The Medical College of Wisconsin's Bioinformatics Research Center designed such a database aimed at storing all this information about source plates. Accordingly, each clone or target DNA is assigned a unique identifier based on its well location and in which plate it is stored on. The database schema is published online at **http://brc.mcw.edu/microarray/components/ clone/DB_design.html.** In practice, even with oligonucleotides, DNA reagents very often need to be transferred from different plate format for carrying out various operations (dilution or concentration, buffer replacement, purification, PCR amplification etc.).

CloneTracker from BioDiscovery and GenePix Pro from Axon Instrument provide a software tool for keeping track of DNA samples during these transfers. The GenePix Pro Plate Converter menu reads a tab delimited text file holding the target DNA identifier arranged in one given format (e.g. 96 well-plate) and writes an output file featuring the new location of the DNA sample with respect to the receiving labware. The scope of CloneTracker encompasses the entire "life cycle" of DNA targets chosen for gridding. It starts from the tracking of sets of DNA samples to the final step of the deposition onto solid support for the array[15]. CloneTracker is especially suited for the manufacture of high density arrays when dealing with numerous sources of DNA samples that need to be arrayed according to various layouts. It reads both a tab delimited file and a database file that hold information about the DNA target identifier with respect to their physical location on the micro-titer labware. The array fabrication workflow takes as arguments at least the number of samples, the format of the micro-titer plate, their number, the destination slide format, the number of pins for gridding, the gridding pattern and the replicate number. All these parameters are setup through the array fabrication user interface. In some instances (e.g. with the Cartesian spotter), these settings can be used directly to program the spotter. They also can be saved for future use. In this respect, CloneTracker can be run as a laboratory information management system (LIMS). It uses a database to monitor the progress of work flowing through the overall array fabrication process. It also assists in controlling the different steps of array fabrication by allowing one to query and update its parameters. Another microarray LIMS has been implemented at the UCSF Ernest Gallo Clinic and Research Center and has been referred to as UC Spots. The rational of the database and its design are posted at **http://www.egcrc.org/bio/ucspots/.** It is comprised of three distinct relational databases which aim to capture information about the PCR cDNA sample preparation procedure, the array fabrication protocol and the data collection procedure respectively. The graphical user interface guides the operator in entering relevant data into the system in order to ensure accurate and exhaustive information for the spotting. UC Spots has been implemented in Java™ which makes it a potent portable application.

Although information systems that keep track of all the accessory data that come with DNA array production are required to ensure the integrity of the data, it is also desirable to think ahead of the fabrication in order to design an exper-iment. A sound design has some impact in the downstream step of raw data pre-processing. One of the pre-processing operations consists of correcting for variability in the background across the array. It is therefore recommended to spread control spots at various locations of the array. Replicates are an effec-tive way to filter out low quality outcome as well as compensate for position effect due notably to the unevenness of the surface of the slide[18, 23]. The third function supplied by CloneTracker is a tool to assist in the design of the microarray. The array design capability allows to forecast the layout of the DNA targets on the slide. The coordinate of any given spot on the array can be locat-ed through the graphical interface. This is achieved through the visual array design interface which offers color-coding for each deriving plate and well loca-tion from a spot on an array. This in silico array design helps to set the grid-ding protocol and ultimately assists in the preparation of the whole experiment.

9.4 DNA Microarray Database Applications

Generating DNA arrays already involves customized data management. Downstream transcription profiling assays are even more demanding in terms of manipulating, sorting and storing rich data sets. When DNA microarray tech-nology emerged as the more relevant approach to assessing transcriptome com-position at a large scale, it became obvious that specific database software is going to be needed. Meanwhile a set of accompanying information was estab-lished[2]. Under the guidance of the international consortium referred to as the Micro Array Gene Expression Databases (MGED, **http://www.mged.org**), a finite set of adequate contextual information was conceived and proposed to the genomics community: this is the MIAME which stands for the Minimum Information About A Microarray Experiment[3]. The explicit motivation was to make gene expression data interchangeable. Unlike DNA or protein sequences, there was   no obvious way of communicating microarray results between research labs. This holds true for the underlying gene expression data as well as for the descriptive data that provide the context for gene expression meas-urement. The data and contextual information that need to be assigned to any gene expression assay have been broken down into the six categories listed below and presented in more details in *Table 9-1*.

1. Experimental design: the set of hybridization experiments in its entirety.

2. Array design: each array used and each element (spot) on the array

3. Samples: samples used, extract preparation and labelling

4. Hybridizations: procedures and parameters

5. Measurements: images, quantification, specifications

6. Normalisation controls: types, values, specifications

These MIAME attributes have reached the consensus of DNA array users and by now are endorsed by journal editors. The six objects defined in the MIAME constitute the foundation for modeling a DNA array database. Accordingly, several software packages have been developed that are making use of this model. In addition, most of DNA array database software include the capability to store and manage gene expression data that have been captured from a different technology platform. These other sources of gene expression data are mainly coming from either macroarray or from high density oligonucleotide array (Affymetrix' exclusive system) or even from the Serial Analysis of Gene Expression technique[28]. A laboratory which is using gene expression data from DNA microarray as well as from other techniques might find it useful to implement a database software able to store data from different sources. Furthermore, a significant amount of SAGE and Affymetrix based data are publicly available and can be readily imported. Therefore, what matters are the system requirements, the MIAME compliance and the commitment into the XML technology. As far as system requirements are concerned, the option is entirely dependent on which database management system the application is expected to run on. Consistent with the Open Source approach, several Academic Institutions have released schema and codes available under the GNU License. These applications can run on Linux which is the Open Source distribution of Unix, use Apache as an HTTP server, Open Source as well and are instances of MySQL which is free if run for nonprofit use (in case the database is planned to perform services, the MySQL instance has to be licensed. Licensing requirements are posted at **www.mysql.com**). Falling into this category is NOMAD that has been developed conjointly between three laboratories at the University of California, San Francisco and Lawrence Berkeley National Laboratory (**http://ucsf-nomad.sourceforge.net/**), GeneX, developed by The National Center for Genome Resources and the Computational Genomics Group at the University of California, Irvine and maxdSQL, designed by the the Microarray group at the University of Manchester (**http://www.bioinf.man.ac.uk/ microarray/maxd/maxdSQL/index.html**). To some extent, the AMAD database which stands for Another MicroArray Database, provides an easy system to implement as it does not require a back end database system. AMAD only requires an Apache server program and is straightforward to install on any Unix distribution. It is particularly suited for laboratories equipped with the Axon Instrument GenePix Pro data acquisition software (Axon Instruments, Inc). AMAD has been developed jointly by Mike Eisen, Max Diehn, Paul Spellman, and

Joseph DeRisi from Stanford University and the University of California (**http://www.microarrays.org/software.html**). However, AMAD and NOMAD are designed to uniquely handle data produced with DNA microarray. Both of them are written in PERL, are queried with an HTTP client application and are optimized to accommodate Axon's GenePix input file. Mike Eisen's AERIE data mining application can read data from both databases. Besides AMAD, the installation of one of the software packages requires to setup the appropriate system environment: this includes a Unix distribution (Red Hat, Debian or Mandrake for Linux), the Apache Web server which is often installed by default, as well as the PERL interpreter (if not, latest versions of Apache HTTP server and PERL interpreter are available at www.apache.org and **http://www.cpan.org/ports/index.html** respectively) and MySQL (**http://www.mysql.com/downloads/index.html**). Thereafter, the AMAD and NOMAD can be downloaded from http://www.microarrays.org/software.html and http://sourceforge.net/projects/ucsf-nomad respectively.

GeneX (**http://www.ncgr.org/genex/**) has been design for handling gene expression data that is based on the common microarray or gene chip data formats. Several tables break up microarray information into a hierarchical data model. An ExperimentSet's table comprises the top level of this structure: it supervises the ArrayMeasurement's table, the sample's table the ArrayLayout's table and the ExperimentSet's table. Altogether, these tables hold information in compliance with MIAME. GeneX has an interesting feature as it distinguishes between the DNA target (the actual sequence that is assayed) and the gene it is supposed to represent. The Canonical Sequence Feature holds the gene sequence whereas the User Sequence Feature field holds the target DNA sequence. GeneX enables XML data exchange. Even though NCGR has defined its own data and data type definition, it will support the standard that is resulting from the Rosetta GEML and the MGED MAML definitions, namely MAGE (**http://www.mged.org/Workgroups/MAGE/mage.html**).

MaxdSQL is an implementation of the ArrayExpress database schema. The SQL codes are ANSI SQL 92 compliant and therefore can be used in either Oracle or MySQL or even PostgreSQL on Linux. MaxdSQL is only available for academics institution. The ArrayExpress database is also supporting the MIAME convention and is breaking up the data into Experiment, Hybridization, Sample, Array and ExpressionValue's tables. The database is queried and uploaded through a Java™ servlet applications referred to as maxdView and maxload. The back-end MaxdSQL service and maxdView and maxload client applications are posted at **http://www.bioinf.man.ac.uk/microarray/resources.html**. GeneDirector™, developed by BioDiscovery, is a comprehensive database management system which fits with CloneTracker as well as ImaGene for array image acquisition and GeneSight for statistical analysis of pre-processing and normalisation output. Based on a relational schema and run above Oracle, these four components constitute the only commercially available fully integrated system.

9.5 DNA microarray Markup Language

In addition to these efforts to standardize the experiments design and the data modifications (preprocessing and normalisation schemes) there is a third and last layer of standardization in order to complete the portability of gene expression data acquired by DNA microarray approaches. It regards the format with which data stored in such dedicated databases will be retrieved. There is a large consensus to adopt a format derived from the eXtensible Markup Language (XML) adapted to a common set of concepts, relations, objects and constraints relative to gene expression data (ontology) which is referred to as MAGE-ML (MicroArray Gene Expression Markup Language)[27]. The MAGE-ML specifications have been recently released (**http://sourceforge.net/ projects/mged/**) and will definitively be the standard as major US and European Institutions are supporting it (mainly Stanford University, the University of Washington in Saint Louis, the WhiteHead Institute, TIGR, NCBI and the European Bioinformatics Institute) as well as Corporations (e.g. Rosetta Inpharmatics). A steering committee has been set-up and is hosted by the EMBL-EBI (the MGED group, Microarray Gene Expression Database - www.mged). The privately launched project lead by Rosetta Inpharmatics, Inc followed by GeneticXchange, InforMax, NetGenics, Agilent, Europroteome AG and Spotfire is merging with the MAGE standard. The project had the same objective (define a file format for exchange and annotation of gene expression) and was referred to as Gene Expression Markup Language (GEML). The authors of GEML and MAML as well as NetGenics are now working together to design a common data structure for communicating microarray based gene expression data.

9.6 Conclusions

Once properly setup, a DNA microarray platform provides a substantial source of data. Admittedly, it involves the management of the resources comprised of the DNA targets in prevision of manufacturing arrays. Down on the line is the requirement of running a data management system which ultimately serves the whole purpose which is to assign expression pattern to gene sequence strings. Notable progress has been recently accomplished in providing software solutions which address the specific needs of DNA array data management. These advancements are making use of the latest information technologies.

Table 9-1

Minimum Information About a Microarray Experiment-MIAME (Version 1.0)

1. Experimental design: the set of hybridisation experiments as a whole

a) author (submitter), laboratory, contact information, links (URL), citations
b) type of the experiment - maximum one line, for instance:

✔ normal vs. diseased comparison
✔ treated vs. untreated comparison
✔ time course
✔ dose response
✔ effect of gene knock-out
✔ effect of gene knock-in (transgenics)

c) experimental variables, i.e. parameters or conditions tested (e.g., time, dose, genetic variation, response to a treatment or compound)
d) single or multiple hybridisations.

For multiple hybridisations:
✔ serial (yes/no)
type (e.g., time course, dose response)
✔ grouping (yes/no)
type (e.g., normal vs. diseased, multiple tissue comparison)

e) quality related indicators, quality control steps taken:

✔ biological replicates?
✔ technical replicates (replicate spots or hybs)?
✔ polyA tails
✔ low complexity regions
✔ unspecific binding
✔ other

f) optional user defined "qualifier, value, source" list (see Introduction)
g) a free text description of the experiment set or a link to a publication

2.1 Array copy (physical instance)

✔ unique ID as used in part 1
✔ array design name

CHAPTER 9
DNA Array Information Workflow and Data Management

Table 9-1 *(continued)*

2.2 Array design

a) array related information

- ✔ array design name (e.g., "Stanford Human 10K set") as given in 2.1
- ✔ platform type: in situ synthesized, spotted or other
- ✔ array provider (source)
- ✔ surface type: glass, membrane, other
- ✔ surface type name
- ✔ physical dimensions of array support (e.g. of slide)
- ✔ number of elements on the array
- ✔ a reference system allowing to locate each element (spot) on the array (in the simplest case the number of columns and rows is sufficient)
- ✔ production date
- ✔ production protocol (obligatory if custom produced)
- ✔ optional "qualifier, value, source" list

b) properties of each type of elements (spots) on the array

- ✔ element type unique ID
- ✔ simple or composite
- ✔ element type: synthetic oligo-nucleotides, PCR products, plasmids, colonies, other
- ✔ single or double stranded
- ✔ element (spot) dimensions
- ✔ element generation protocol that includes sufficient information to reproduce the element
- ✔ attachment (covalent/ionic/other)
- ✔ optional "qualifier, value, source" list

c) specific properties of each element (spot) on the array: element type ID from 2.2b

- ✔ clone ID, clone provider, date, availability
- ✔ sequence or PCR primer information:
- ✔ sequence accession number in DDBJ/EMBL/GenBank if known
- ✔ sequence itself (if databases do not contain it)
- ✔ primer pair information, if relevant
- ✔ for composite oligonucleotide elements:

Table 9-1 *(continued)*

✔ oligonucleotide sequences, if given
✔ number of oligonucleotides and the reference sequence
(or accession number), otherwise

3. Samples: samples used, extract preparation and labeling

a) sample source and treatment ID as used in section 1organism (NCBI taxonomy) additional "qualifier, value, source" list; each qualifier in the list is obligatory if applicable; the list includes:

✔ cell source and type (if derived from primary sources (s))
✔ sex
✔ age
✔ growth conditions
✔ development stage
✔ organism part (tissue)
✔ animal/plant strain or line
✔ genetic variation (e.g. gene knockout transgenic variation)
✔ individual
✔ individual genetic characteristics (e.g. disease allele polymorphisms)
✔ disease state or normal
✔ target cell type
✔ cell line and source (if applicable)
✔ in vivo treatments (organism or individual treatments)
✔ in vitro treatments (cell culture conditions)
✔ treatment type (e.g. small molecule heat shock cold shock food deprivation)
✔ compound
✔ is additional clinical information available (link)
✔ separation technique (e.g., none, trimming, microdissection, FACS) laboratory protocol for sample treatment

b) hybridisation extract preparation

✔ extraction method
✔ whether total RNA, mRNA, or genomic DNA is extracted
✔ amplification (RNA polymerases, PCR)
✔ optional "qualifier, value, source" list
✔ labeling
✔ ID as given in section 1

Table 9-1 *(continued)*

✔ laboratory protocol for labelling, including
✔ amount of nucleic acids labeled
✔ label used (e.g., A-Cy3, G-Cy5, 33P, ...)
✔ label incorporation method
✔ optional "qualifier, value, source" list

4. Hybridisations: procedures and parameters

✔ ID as given in section 1
✔ laboratory protocol for hybridisation, including:
✔ the solution (e.g., concentration of solutes)
✔ blocking agent
✔ wash procedure
✔ quantity of labelled target used
✔ time, concentration, volume, temperature
✔ description of the hybridisation instruments
✔ optional "qualifier, value, source" list

5. Measurements: images, quantitation, specifications:
hybridisation scan raw data:

a1) the scanner image file (e.g., TIFF, DAT) from the hybridised microarray scanning
a2) scanning information:

✔ input: hybridisation ID as in Section 1
✔ image unique ID
✔ scan parameters, including laser power, spatial resolution, pixel space, PMT voltage;
✔ laboratory protocol for scanning, including:
✔ scanning hardware
✔ scanning software
✔ image analysis and quantitation

b1) the complete image analysis output (of the particular image analysis software) for each element (or composite element - see 2.2.b), for each channel
b2) image analysis information:

✔ input: image ID
✔ quantitation unique ID

Table 9-1 *(continued)*

✔ image analysis software specification and version, availability, and the description or identification of the algorithm

c1) derived measurement value summarizing related elements as used by the author (this may constitute replicates of the element on the same or different arrays or hybridisations, as well as different elements related to the same entity e.g., gene)

c2) reliability indicator for the value of c1) as used by the author (e.g., standard deviation); may be "unknown"

c3) specification how c1 and c2 are calculated

✔ input: one or more quantitation ID's

6.Normalisation controls, values, specifications

✔ Normalisation strategy
✔ spiking
✔ "housekeeping" genes
✔ total array
✔ optional user defined "quality value"
✔ Normalisation algorithm
✔ linear regression
✔ log-linear regression
✔ ratio statistics
✔ log(ratio) mean/median centering
✔ nonlinear regression
✔ optional user defined "quality value"
✔ Control array elements
✔ position (the abstract coordinate on the array)
✔ control type (spiking, normalization, negative, positive)
✔ control qualifier (endogenous, exogenous)
✔ optional user defined "quality value"
✔ Hybridisation extract preparation
✔ spike type
✔ spike qualifier
✔ target element
✔ optional user defined "quality value"

Acknowledgement

The author gratefully acknowledge Dr. Laszlo Takacs and Dr. Alexander Kuklin for their valuable assistance in writing this manuscript.

Reference

1. *Adams et al.* : The genome sequence of Drosophila melanogaster. *Science* 2000 :2185-2195.

2. *Brazma A*: On the importance of standardisation in life sciences. *Bioinformatics 2001*; 17:113-114

3. *Brazma A, Hingamp P, Quackenbush J, Sherlock G, Spellman P, Stoeckert C, Aach J, Ansorge W, Ball CA, Causton HC, Gaasterland T, Glenisson P, Holstege FC, Kim IF, Markowitz V, Matese JC, Parkinson H, Robinson A, Sarkans U, Schulze-Kremer S, Stewart J, Taylor R, Vilo J, Vingron M*: Minimum information about a microarray experiment (MIAME) - toward standards for microarray data. *Nat Genet 2001*; 4:365-371.

4. *Brenner S, Johnson M, Bridgham J, Golda G, Lloyd DH, Johnson D, Luo S, McCurdy S, Foy M, Ewan M, Roth R, George D, Eletr S, Albrecht G, Vermaas E, Williams SR, Moon K, Burcham T, Pallas M, DuBridge RB, Kirchner J, Fearon K, Mao J, Corcoran K*: Gene expression analysis by massively parallel signature sequencing (MPSS) on microbead arrays. *Nat Biotechnol 2000*; 18: 630-634

5. *Burge C and Karlin S*: Prediction of complete gene structures in human genomic DNA. *J Mol Biol* 1997; 268:78-94.

6. *Davenport RJ*: Microarrays. Data standards on the horizon. *Science 2001*; 292:414-5

7. *Duggan DJ, Bittner M, Chen Y, Meltzer P, Trent JM*: Expression profiling using cDNA microarays. *Nat Genet Supplement* 1999; 21: 10-14.

8. *Dunaeva M, Adamska I*: Identification of genes expressed in response to light stress in leaves of Arabidopsis thaliana using RNA differential display. *Eur J Biochem* 2001; 268:5521-5529.

9. *Iyer VR, Eisen MB, Ross DT, Schuler G, Moore T, Lee JCF, Trent JM, Staudt LM, Hudson Jr J, Boguski MS, Lashkari D, Shalon D, Botstein D, Brown P*: The transcriptional program in the response of human fibroblasts to serum. *Science 1999*; 283: 83-87.

10. *Jia L, Young MF, Powell J, Yang L, Ho NC, Hotchkiss R, Robey PG, Francomano CA*. Gene expression profile of human bone marrow stromal cells: high-throughput expressed sequence tag sequencing analysis. *Genomics 2002*; 79:7-17.

11. *Jiang C, Lu H, Vincent KA, Shankara S, Belanger AJ, Cheng SH, Akita GY, Kelly RA, Goldberg MA, Gregory RJ*: Gene expression profiles in human cardiac cells subjected to hypoxia or expressing a hybrid form of HIF-1{alpha}. *Physiol Genomics 2002*; 11:23-32.

12. *Kalocsai P, Shams S*: Use of bioinformatics in arrays. *Methods Mol Biol* 2001; 170:223-236.

13. *Korf I, Flicek P, Duan D, Brent MR*: Integrating genomic homology into gene structure prediction. *Bioinformatics 2001*; 17 :S140-148.

14. *Kowalczuk M, Mackiewicz P, Gierlik A, Dudek MR, Cebrat S*: Total number of coding open reading frames in the yeast genome. *Yeast* 1999; 15:1031-1034.

15. *Kuklin A and Smith J*: DNA array experimental design and databasing with CloneTracker. 2000; *BioDiscovery, Inc.* Los Angeles, CA.

16. *Kuklin A, Shah S, Hoff B and Shams S*: Information processing issues and solutions associated with microarray technology. *LRA 2000*; 12:317-327.

17. *Lander et al.* : International Human Genome Sequencing Consortium. Initial sequencing and analysis of the human genome. *Nature 2001*; 409:860-921.

18. *Lee M-L T, Kuo F C., Whitmore G A and Sklar J*: Importance of replication in microarray gene expression studies: statistical methods and evidence from repetitive cDNA hybridizations. *Proc Natl Acad Sci USA* 2000; 97:9834-9839.

19. *Liu R, States DJ*: Consensus promoter identification in the human genome utilizing expressed gene markers and gene modeling. *Genome Res.* 2000 12:462-469.

20. *Lipshutz RJ, Fodor SPA, Gingeras TR, Lockhart DJ*: High density synthetic oligonucleotide arrays. *Nature Gen Supplement* 1999 21: 20-23.

21. *Ludwig MZ, Bergman C, Patel NH, Kreitman M.* Evidence for stabilizing selection in a eukaryotic enhancer element. *Nature 2000*; 403:564-567.

22. *Novichkov PS, Gelfand MS, Mironov AA*: Gene recognition in eukaryotic DNA by comparison of genomic sequences. *Bioinformatics 2001*; 17:1011-108

23. *Ochs MF and Bidaut G* : Microarray Data Normalization. In Shah S and Kamberova G (eds): Microarray Image Analysis - Nuts & Bolts. Abington, *DNA Press*, 2002.

24. *Perou CM, Jeffrey SS, van de Rijn M, Rees CA, Eisen MB, Ross DT, Pergamenschikov A, Williams CF, Zhu SX, Lee JC, Lashkari D, Shalon D, Brown PO, Botstein D*: Distinctive gene expression patterns in human mammary epithelial cells and breast cancers. *Proc Natl Acad Sci U S A* 1999; 96:9212-9217.

25. *Rajeevan MS, Ranamukhaarachchi DG, Vernon SD, Unger ER*: Use of real-time quantitative PCR to validate the results of cDNA array and differential display PCR technologies. *Methods* 2001; 25:443-451.

26. *Rocha D, Carrier A, Naspetti M, Victorero G, Anderson E, Botcherby M, Guenet JL, Nguyen C, Naquet P, Jordan BR*: Modulation of mRNA levels in the presence of thymocytes and genome mapping for a set of genes expressed in mouse thymic epithelial cells. *Immunogenetics* 1997; 46:142-151.

27. *Spellman PT*: The future of publishing microarray data. *Brief Bioinform* 2001; 2:316-318.

28. *Stoeckert C, Pizarro A, Manduchi E, Gibson M, Brunk B, Crabtree J, Schug J,Shen-Orr S, Overton GC*: A relational schema for both array-based and SAGE gene expression experiments. *Bioinformatics* 2001;17:300-308.

29. *Tanay VA, Tancowny BP, Glencorse TA, Bateson AN*: The quantitative analysis of multiple mRNA species using oligonucleotide probes in an S1 nuclease protection assay. *Mol Biotechnol* 1997; 7:217-229.

30. *The Washington University Genome Sequencing Center*. Genome sequence of the nematode C. elegans: a platform for investigating biology. The C. elegans Sequencing Consortium. *Science* 1998; 282 :2012-2018.

31. *Yue H, Eastman PS, Wang BB, Minor J, Doctolero MH, Nuttall RL, Stack R, Becker JW, Montgomery JR, Vainer M, Johnston R*: An evaluation of the performance of cDNA microarrays for detecting changes in global mRNA expression. *Nucleic Acids Res* 2001; 29:E41-1

BAC MICROARRAYS

S. Shah, J.P. Gregg[2], M. Mohammed[1], W. Yu[1], S. Damani[1] *and* R.C. Locker[1]

[1] *Spectral Genomics, Inc., Houston, TX USA*
[2] *University of California, Davis School of Medicine, Davis, CA USA*

Contact:
Mansoor Mohammed, Ph.D.
Spectral Genomics, Inc., 8080 North Stadium Drive, Houston, Texas 77054 U.S.A.
E-mail: mmohammed@spectralgenomics.com

0-9664027-5-8/02/$0.00+$.50   *From:* **Microarray Image Analysis-Nuts & Bolts** (pp.185-202)
©2002 by DNA Press, LLC   Edited by: S. Shah and G. Kamberova

10.1 Introduction

Over the last several years there has been an explosion of microarray technology in the biosciences, medical sciences, biotechnology, and pharmaceutical industry. The technology has centered on providing a platform for determining the gene expression profiles of hundreds to tens of thousands of genes (or transcript levels of RNA species) in tissue, tumors, cells, or biological fluids in a single experiment. The rapid and global adoption of this technology has been predicated on its simplicity and success in providing large amounts of highly relevant data.

In their most generic form, microarrays are ordered sets of DNA molecules attached to a solid surface as discussed in Chapter 1 of this book. The DNA molecules are typically either oligonucleotide (ranging form 35 base pairs to several hundred) or cDNAs. The matrix to which the DNA molecule is attached is usually glass, silicon, or nylon. The DNA is attached to the matrix in an ordered pattern such that hundreds to tens of thousands of DNA molecules may be spotted. With this ordered set of DNA segments attached to the surface, RNA from a specimen (e.g. tissue, cell line, tumor) can be either directly or indirectly labeled (usually with a fluorescent nucleotide) and hybridized to the array of genes. The amount of fluorescence at each DNA spot corresponds to the transcript level of that particular gene. Therefore, the expression of thousands of genes can be analyzed in a single specimen.

Microarrays have been exploited for gene expression studies but other applications can be envisioned and developed. One such application is the use of microarrays to study genomic DNA for gains and losses of chromosomal regions, which is the subject of this chapter.

As our understanding of the sequence, structure and function of the human genome increases, fluctuations in DNA sequence copy number with concomitant microscopic or cryptic chromosomal aberrations are becoming increasingly correlated with phenotypic abnormalities[1, 2, 3, 4, 5]. This is particularly important in medicine as many diseases, cancers, and syndromes are caused by deletions, amplifications, and duplication of DNA segments. Classic examples include the deletion of 15q11.2 in Prader-Wili Syndrome[6], trisomy 21 in Down's syndrome[7], and the amplification of erbB2 in breast cancer[8]. In cancer biology, the development of most solid tumors follows a defined series of histopathological stages, involving multiple genetic changes such as translocations, deletions, duplications and alterations in ploidy (chromosomal copy number changes).

Constitutional changes in DNA sequence copy number have now been well documented for a number of genetic syndromes, while acquired changes are receiving tremendous attention by virtue of their association with neoplastic transformations. One of the ultimate aims of genetic testing, therefore, has been to provide as complete as possible a genome-wide analysis for the detection of these fluctuations in DNA sequence copy number so as to facilitate the clinician's predictive, diagnostic or prognostic decisions regarding the disease state of a patient. Traditionally, depending on the nature of the genetic material to be analyzed, chromosomes or total genomic DNA, the genetic testing would be routed to one of two primary laboratories, either a clinical cytogenetics or a molecular diagnostic laboratory. Chromosome analysis were the hallmark of the clinical cytogenetics laboratory while DNA analysis were more often viewed as a substrate for molecular diagnostics. However, with the advancements in molecular cytogenetic diagnostics within the last decade and more recently the completion of the draft sequence of the human genome, this demarcation has become increasingly permeated.

Over the last decade, techniques have been developed to study chromosomal number and DNA copy number. Classical cytogenetics has been used for decades to karyotype cells (number and classification of the chromosomes in a cell) but is limited due to the need to culture the cells, make metaphase chromosomes, and requires expertise in interpreting the chromosomal spreads. In addition, cytogenetics only provides a crude analysis of the chromosome number and has little sensitivity in identifying deletions and amplifications. In order to address these limitations of classical cytogenetics, high-resolution cytogenetics and now-classical chromosomal genomic hybridization (CGH) have been developed. These techniques suffer from the same technical difficulties of classic cytogenetics and still provide limited chromosomal resolution (>5 Mb).

Novel techniques such as whole chromosome painting probes (WCPP)[9]; reverse chromosome painting, multiplex chromosome coloring[10], and subtelomeric chromosome labeling[11, 12] have shown considerable promise for the identification of some subtle rearrangements. However, neither of these techniques are uniquely suited for the purpose, they all suffer limitations, and their ability to detect small aberrations remains uncertain. WCPP are not amenable for use in routine screening, because (1) they exclude significant tracts in the subtelomeric regions where cryptic aberrations may occur, and (2) the assay cannot be completed in a single experiment using one slide, due to the inability to simultaneously paint all chromosomes. Even in the case of multiplex FISH, the sensitivity for detecting cryptic aberrations is presently unknown[13]. Therefore, with current technology, there is great potential to miss disease-associated smaller "cryptic" chromosomal deletions or amplifications, some of which may have been systematically undetected.

The introduction of comparative genomic hybridization (CGH) to metaphase chromosomes revolutionized the clinical cytogenetics diagnostic arena by permitting the genome wide analysis of cancer specimens with chromosomal aberrations that were either too many or too complex to be fully characterized by routine cytogenetics[14]. Moreover, since CGH required only genomic DNA from the specimen sample, it permitted the analysis of specimens from which chromosomal preparations were either impractical or impossible. In addition, it introduced genomic DNA as a substrate for analysis to the clinical cytogenetics laboratory. However, the use of metaphase chromosomes as the platform against which the CGH was performed meant that the inherent resolution levels associated with metaphase chromosomes persisted. In practice, this meant that CGH to metaphase chromosomes remained largely incapable of accomplishing genome-wide screens for chromosomal aberrations that were less than about 5 Mb, a limitation which made this approach unsuitable for detecting many of the non-cancer-related genetic aberrations encountered in the routine day-to-day portfolio of a clinical cytogenetics laboratory.

The advent of BAC array technology and the ability to screen the entire genome have re-drawn the attention to the applicability of CGH, albeit array CGH, in the routine cytogenetics laboratory. So-called array or matrix CGH utilizes mapped DNA sequences in a microarray format as an alternative platform for the CGH analysis. Hence, the resolution level of this approach is dependent on a combination of the number, size and map positions of the DNA elements within the array. Several reports have described adaptation of microarray technology to the study of genomic alterations[4,15]. Unfortunately, these technologies have been difficult to adapt to clinical and research laboratories.

The introduction of commercial BAC arrays (Spectral Genomics, Inc.), which are manufactured under strict robust processes, has yielded high-resolution genomic scans (at the time of this writing 1 Mb) in a rapid and highly reproducible fashion. We have begun testing the suitability of the BAC array approach with commercially available human genome arrays for incorporation into the day-to-day repertoire of cytogenetic diagnostic procedures. A number of clinical specimens as well as cell lines with a broad spectrum of known constitutional and acquired genetic aberrations were chosen for the study, the results of which, conclusively demonstrate the evolving position of microarray genome profiling as an indispensable addition to the repertoire of cytogenetic diagnostic procedures. In this chapter, we will discuss BAC array technology with a stronger focus on the experimental design, image analysis and data normalization.

10.2 Genome Wide Molecular Pathology Approaches

Several research programs are underway, which should provide a better understanding of the gene expression profiles of tumor cells under the direction of the NCI funded Cancer Genome Anatomy Project (CGAP). Although the information provided by this strategy will ultimately be valuable in defining key molecular components required for the proliferation of a cancer cell, a mammoth experimental effort is required to understand the expression profile of a single tumor by this methodology. This approach is burdensome as many of the genes identified as differentially expressed may not be directly responsible for the pathology or disease; rather they may be innocent bystanders. However, by sifting through this information, it may be possible to identify some diagnostic indicators (expressed genes) of certain pathological states and these may ultimately be useful clinically. For example, serum markers such as PSA are used to monitor the progression of prostate tumors and markers such as the expression of estrogen receptor are used clinically to ascertain whether a tumor should be treated with preventive agents like tamoxifen. Antibody based therapy has been approved for breast tumors which express the marker her2/neu. It is important to point out that tumors are typically screened for just a handful of markers, as a result clinical treatments are usually performed relatively blind with respect to the genetic characteristics of the tumor.

10.3 Limitations of Gene Expression Arrays

Although there is great interest in using expression arrays, it is now possible to screen the genome of a sample or tumor for genomic changes (gains and losses of DNA), as an alternative to the examination of transcriptional activity of a cell or tissue. Analysis of the genome offers several advantages over the examination of mRNA levels; namely it is less variable than alterations in the relative message levels of the approximate 30,000 human genes[16,17]. This reduced complexity greatly simplifies the identification of causal genetic changes in individuals and tumors. A second advantage is that the locus-to-locus variation is small, either allele loss (50 to 100% signal loss) or locus amplification (up to 100 fold). Thus the dynamic range of analysis is likely to be much more manageable for obtaining a relevant readout across a large number of samples.

In addition, there are several limitations of expression microarrays but mainly; *it is difficult to discriminating cause from effect*. Messenger RNAs are present at many different levels in a cell/tissue and typically vary over several orders of magnitude. Looking for the most prominent expression level changes in a tumor or sample will be biased for those genes abundantly expressed in one of the two samples; therefore, it is quite difficult to know what a "significant" expression level of a gene actually is. Is a 1.5 fold change important or is a

100-fold change more important? The answer is speculative but demonstrates the difficulty in interpreting gene expression arrays.

10.4 Comparative Genomic Hybridization (CGH)

The genome is a far better place to define the genetic changes in germline lymphocyte and tumors samples than in any other sample. Changes in the genome are the cause rather than the *effect* of neoplastic growth. Compared with the transcribed genome there is much less stochastic "noise" and thus key relevant prognostic changes can be identified. In the past, the analysis of the genomes of tumors has been accomplished with the process of comparative genomic hybridization (CGH) of fluorescently labeled DNA to metaphase spreads described in Figure 10-1[18,19]. In this well refined technique, genomic DNA from the tumor is labeled with a fluorescent dye in one color while a normal reference sample is labeled in a different color and these sample are co-hybridized to normal metaphase spreads. Chromosomal imbalances across the genome in the test (tumor) DNA sample are quantified and positionally defined by analyzing the ratio of fluorescence of the two different colors along the target metaphase chromosomes. CGH has been successfully applied to analyze a variety of human tumors to detect chromosomal imbalances[20]. However, the resolution of CGH applied to metaphase spreads is limited by cytogenetic resolution, namely several megabases (~5 Mb), and considerable cytogenetics expertise is required to apply this method, especially in other mammalian species. Given that chromosome distribution in every metaphase spread is unique, it is very hard to develop automated methods for data capture and analysis. Moreover, the use of metaphase spreads limits the sensitivity of the method. CGH performed on metaphase spreads is therefore not a high throughput technology and is limited to specialist research applications.

10.5 Bacterial Artificial Chromosomes (BACs) Arrays

Over the last several years, BAC arrays have been described and can used to circumvent the considerable limitations of CGH and chromosome spreads while maintaining the power of a full genome scan. Instead of spotting an oligonucleotide or PCR amplified cDNA product, as done in gene expression arrays, Bacterial Artificial Chromosomes (BACs) are spotted onto an ordered array. BACs are large-insert DNA clones that have been cytogenetically and physically mapped to the human genome. Currently, over 8,800 large-insert clones (BACs represent the majority of these clones) have been mapped to the human genome, with at least one clone on average per megabase (Mb) for 23 of the 24 chromosomes, and clone density ranging from greater than 5 clones per Mb for chromosomes 1, 6, 20, 22 and X to about 0.3 clones per Mb for chromosome Y[21,22]. This resource affords the opportunity to use these BACs to generate an ordered array of DNA segments at a very high genomic resolution.

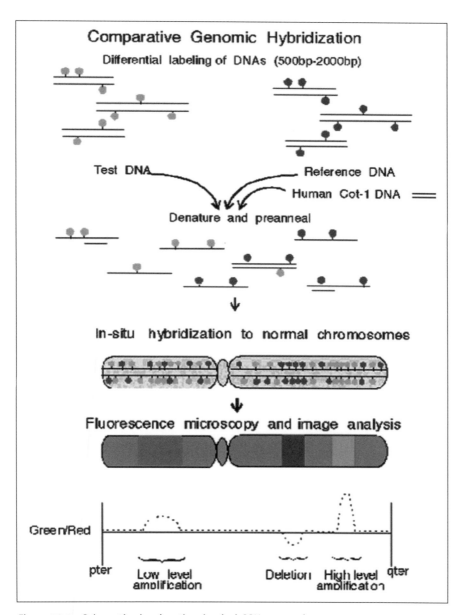

Figure 10-1. Schematic showing the classical CGH approach.

Therefore, the limitations on classical CGH are avoided by replacing metaphase spreads as the hybridization template with micro-arrays of cloned DNA (BACs), which are covalently coupled onto glass microscope slides. For example, genomic DNA from a normal sample (karyotypicaly normal germline DNA) is labeled with Cy5 (a fluorescent dye) and genomic DNA from test sample (tumor or patient) is labeled with Cy3 (a different fluorescent dye); these labeled samples are co-hybridized to arrays of BAC clones on glass microscope slides. A high-resolution fluorescent scanner captures the fluorescent intensity of the array and converts intensities of the fluorescence signals into an intensity ratio histogram. The fluorescence ratio of the two colors can be compared between different spots representing different genomic regions. This provides a genome-wide molecular profile of the sample with respect to regions of the genome that are deleted or amplified, compared with the normal genome, at the resolution of a BAC (200 kb). The overall approach is summarized in Figure 10-2.

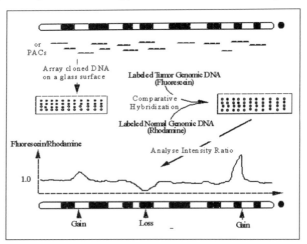

Figure 10-2. Comparative hybridization on cloned DNA to detect chromozomal imbalances.

Array CGH has several significant advantages over metaphase CGH:

1. The signal intensity is enhanced, since the hybridization targets are multiple-copy cloned DNA, not a single DNA molecule.

2. The resolution can be greatly increased—to size of the target clone (BAC) on the array (about 200 kb).

3. The method can be automated, enabling the entire genome of many tumors to be screened in a single assay.

10.6 Technical Challenges for Genomic Arrays

As the conceptual use of BAC arrays has been obvious, there have been technical challenges that have needed to be addressed before these arrays could become commonplace. Traditional DNA microarrays are limited in the size of fragment that can be attached to the matrix. Most microarrays are made either with short oligonucleotides or with PCR amplified cDNA fragments. One of the main difficulties in producing large insert DNA arrays/BAC arrays has been the attachment of the DNA and its availability for hybridization. Traditional techniques for attaching DNA to a solid surface rely on derivatizing the slide surface such that it has available activated or functional groups for chemically or covalently attaching a DNA segment. This process has had varying degrees of success, but better technology was needed for BAC arrays and this has proved to be strategic limitation for the application of BAC arrays.

Spectral Genomics has developed an innovative twist to the attachment chemistry. Instead of treating and functionally-activating the solid surface, the DNA molecule is chemically modified and functionally activated. This allows for more robust attachment and decreased background. The modified nucleic acid is comprised of a nucleic acid covalently bound to a moiety containing two crucial functional groups: a cyclic ether group and an alkoxysilane group. Many of the advantages seen in this technology are derived from the fact that the solid surface, typically ordinary glass, remains highly chemically inert. Thus, the common problems of probe binding non-specifically to the glass, as well as the spreading of targets are eliminated. The final result is that, among other things, there is higher sensitivity of detection compared with the state-of-the-art derivatized solid support. In addition, the nucleic acid to be immobilized upon the solid support is readily derivatized. The reaction of the epoxide derivatives occurs under mild conditions, reaction rates are quick, and equilibrium is maintained. Moreover, the epoxide-modified nucleic acid is permanently stable. The chemistry is also very flexible. Nucleotides are not the only molecules that can be attached to the matrix and the matrix does not have to be a glass slide. For instance, as the machines to scan beads become more prevalent, microarrays on beads (fluid arrays) can also be offered. Finally, the novel attachment chemistry is ideally suited for attaching long fragments of DNA to the matrix. Thus, a whole new area of genome scanning is opened up for novel applications.

10.7 BAC Array Experimental Design and Image Analysis

In a typical BAC array experiment, random priming (Klenow fragment) is used to label isolated genomic DNA. For each experiment, the sample is labeled with Cy3 in one reaction, Cy5 in another reaction, while the control is also labeled with Cy3 and Cy5 in separate reactions (see *Panel 10A* for outline of the protocol). By labeling the sample and control with both Cy3 and Cy5, the dye reversal experiments can be conducted. This is necessary due to the differential incorporation efficiencies of the Cy3 and Cy5 dyes, as well as their differences in fluorescent stability. The slide is then immediately scanned.

Panel 10A:
Outline of Genomic DNA Labeling Protocol for Use with BAC Microparrays

- 1 µg each of test and reference DNA is fragmented by either brief sonication or overnight restriction enzyme digestion (such as with EcoR I).

- The fragmented DNA is then denatured in the presence of random primers by boiling for 5 min.

- A labeling buffer comprising of dNTPs, 1mM Cy3-dCTP or Cy5-dCTP and Klenow fragment is then added to the sample DNA and the mixture is incubated at 37°C for 1-2 hr.

- The labeled test and control DNAs (test-Cy3 and control-Cy5, and the converse), as well as Cot-1 blocking DNA, are mixed and precipitated together.

- The pellet is dissolved in a formamide/dextran sulfate based hybridization buffer, denatured at 72°C for 10 min, snap-cooled on ice and incubated at 37°C for 30 min.

- The labeled DNA solution is then placed on the center of the array, covered with a cover-slip and the array is hybridized overnight (15-20 hr) at 37°C in a humidity-controlled hybridization chamber.

- A post-hybridization wash of the array is performed at 50°C in 2X SSC, 50% formamide for 20 min and is repeated with 2X SSC, 0.1% NP-40 and with 0.2X SSC. A final brief wash with double distilled water is performed and the slides are spun dried and stored desiccated in the dark until scanning.

The BAC arrays are scanned on a two-color fluorescent scanner, creating two 16-bit TIFF images. The images are downloaded from the scanner and analyzed using a commercial software program (SpectralWare™ from Spectral Genomics, Inc.). The software program automatically detects the regions of fluorescent signal, determine signal intensity, and compile the data into an Excel spreadsheet that is linked to clone name, position in the genome, and the duplicate clone position. SpectralWare has a module that normalizes the Cy3/Cy5 intensity ratios for each slide and each data point. In particular, each slide is globally normalized such that the summed Cy3 signal equals the summed Cy5 signal. In order for a BAC to be identified as a significantly differentially represented, the fluorescent intensity of the BAC duplicates are averaged and must show a change greater than two standard deviations (SD) over the normal control. This then has to be reproduced in the dye reversal experiment in order for the data point to be categorized as significantly differentially represented. The software then compiles the data to generate chromosome plots. In addition, the software creates a tab-delimited file of the data including the raw data, normalized data, and statistics showing copy change.

Therefore, BAC arrays rely on simple principles; collect a DNA sample from patient and an unaffected individual, label them with different dyes and hybridize to the microarray. Scanning of the hybridized arrays results in images that can be automatically analyzed by the software system. Replicate clones on the arrays provide a high confidence evaluation of the copy number of each DNA segment. The availability of these microarrays, associated protocols, and software system not only reduces the need for highly skilled personnel, but gives the laboratory the ability for high-volume sample analysis without resulting increases in workload, and ultimately potential the realization of significant cost savings.

10.8 Data transformations and normalizations for BAC arrays

The key information that needs to be recorded from microarrays is the intensity strength of each target/clone. Given the comparative nature of these studies, one is typically interested in the difference in intensity levels between the test and reference populations. This translates to differences in the function of intensities on the two images, each generated by one dye. Under idealized conditions, the total florescent intensity from a spot is proportional to the number of copies of the DNA sequence present in the hybridized sample. Given the noise variations in array experiments, these idealized conditions are never met. In order to compensate for noise variations, an estimate of noise signal is typically subtracted from the spot signal.

The common values computed are for the spot signal and noise signal are total, mean, median, mode, volume, intensity ratio, and the correlation ratio across two channels as discussed in previous chapters of this book. The underlying principle for judging which one is the best method, is based on how well each of these measurements correlates to the amount of the DNA probe present at each spot location. In particular, each slide will be globally normalized such that the summed Cy3 signal equals the summed Cy5 signal. In order for a BAC to be identified as a significantly differentially represented, the fluorescent intensity of the BAC duplicates are averaged and must show a change greater than two standard deviations (SD) over the normal control. This then has to be reproduced in the dye reversal experiment in order for the data point to be categorized as significantly differentially represented. One can then compile the data to generate chromosome profiles.

In the analysis of chromosome 13 arrays, the median signal value of pixels around each spot was subtracted from the median signal value of each spot. A fixed distance of 5 pixels from the periphery of each spot was used to calculate the background intensity values. Each of background subtracted values can now be used to compute the ratio of the two channels. By dividing the intensity value of the sample by the control, one can estimate the ratio of sequences present in the sample over the control.

The next important step is to normalize the data. Various dyes used in array studies produce different results due to different biochemical properties. Due to his inherent bias, it is critical to perform normalization of the two channels to accurately estimate the ratio value, which in effect reflects the changes in DNA sequence copies. The idea of a flip dye experiment is introduced to control such phenomena. Let us assume that the first experiment, also referred to as the forward experiment, has the control labeled with Cy3 and the treatment sample labeled with Cy5. We will calculate the ratio of the two channels as:

$$R_1 = Cy5_1 \, / \, Cy3_1$$

Similarly, ratio of the the flip dye experiment, or the reverse experiment, is given by:

$$R_2 = Cy3_2 \, / \, Cy5_2$$

A plot of intensity signals registered on the two channels for the same DNA should produce a straight line $Cy3_1 = Cy5_2$ and $Cy3_2 = Cy5_1$. Accepting small random variations from the normal reference line, the general trend indicates a non-negligible influence that should be corrected. Similar expectations hold for experiments involving most of the genome as it is assumed that most sequences will not change.

The final normalization step tries to obtain values that are independent of the experiment and hopefully can be compared with other values. This is achieved by applying an iterative linear regression, where the regression is performed, residuals are identified, spots having residuals greater than 2 standard deviations away from the mean ratio are neglected, regression is applied again to the remainder of the values, and the procedure repeated until the residuals become less than a fixed threshold. The same normalization is applied to both of the dye flip experiments. Hence, the above procedure cross-normalizes the two dye flip experiments and then performs an inter-experiment normalization.

The next step is to perform the analysis of the replicate spots on the array. In order to statistically combine the replicates, one has to estimate the probability distribution of the normalized ratios. Due to the non-linear behavior of the dyes over extended intensity ranges, many earlier methods have assumed that the ratios are not distributed normally, but that taking the logarithm of the ratios provides a closer estimate to a normal distribution. There are several reasons for doing the above. Firstly, the log makes the distribution symmetrical. Let us consider the ratio values 1, 10, and 100. If one considers the difference between the middle values and the two extremes, one is tempted to consider the difference to the right more important than the difference to the left. However, from a biological point of view, the phenomenon is the same, namely there is a ten copy change in both cases. The log transforms the values into log(1), log(10), and log(100) which is 0, 1, and 2, reflecting the fact than the phenomena are the same. The second advantage is that the log decouples the variance and the mean intensity and makes the distribution normal. Replicates can now be combined by calculating mean, median, or mode and the coefficients of variance(cv). This produces the so-called average-log-ratios.

While the advantages of symmetrical scaling is true for expression estimation, it does not hold true for estimating genomic sequence copies, as is the case with genomic arrays. The sequence changes exhibit a much smaller dynamic range, and copy change in thousands is never the case. Hence, in our estimation, we calculate the skewness of the both the normalized ratios and the log normalized ratios to estimate the parameters of the distribution. In the event of normalized ratios being normally distributed, one can easily calculate the mean and variance. If the skewness factor indicates that the log normalized ratios are normally distributed, we estimate:

$$f(R|\mu,\sigma^2) = \frac{1}{2\pi\sigma^2}\, e^{-(\log r - \mu)^2 / 2\sigma^2}$$

where,

$$ER = e^{\mu + (\sigma^2/2)} \; ; \; VarR = e^{2(\mu+\sigma^2)} - e^{2\mu+\sigma^2}$$

Given, r_1 and r_2, replicates ratios of the same clone, we can estimate the mean and variance as:

$$\mu_r = \frac{r_1 - r_2}{2} \; ; \; \sigma_r^2 = (r_1 - \mu_r)^2 + (r_2 - \mu_r)^2$$

This leads to the estimation of a single combined mean value of the two replicates as well as the variance for the mean of the two replicates.

The final step in estimating the ratio value for each sequence on the array is to combine the ratio estimates of the flip dye experiments. Though the two experiments have been normalized, the variance within each experiment is different. If $M_{R_1}(t)$ and $M_{R_2}(t)$ are the moment generating functions for the two distributions, r_1 and r_2 are the ratio values for the same clones from each of the experiments, the combined estimate is given by

$$r_c = \frac{r_1 + r_2}{2}.$$

Thus, the new distribution can be estimated by

$$M_{R_c}(t) = \frac{M_{R_1}(t)M_{R_2}(t)}{2}.$$

This allows us to calculate the variance of the combined ratio as

$$\sigma^2_{r_c} = \frac{\sigma^2_{r_1} + \sigma^2_{r_2}}{2}.$$

10.9 Sensitivity and Reproducability with BAC Arrays

In order to demonstrate the sensitivity, reproducibility, and specificity of BAC arrays, we performed a pilot study to evaluate the current version of human BAC arrays from Spectral Genomics. These BAC arrays allow the entire human genome to be viewed simultaneously at a 3Mb resolution. The goal in the first experiment was to analyze the sensitivity that will allow the detection of single copy changes as well as to test the detection of gene dosage difference between normal male and female DNA.

In this study, we conducted a normal male-to-male hybridization and a normal male-to-female hybridization. We repeated both the experiments five times, and each hybridization was repeated by reversing the dye incorporation in each sample so as to capture variations from one array to another. Cyanine dyes (Cy3 and Cy5) were used to label the male and female genomic DNA using random priming. After hybridizing at 37°C for 16 hours, imaging was performed using the GenePix 4000A laser scanner from Axon, Inc., and the images were analyzed using the SpectralWare system (Spectral Genomics, Inc.).

Figure 3 shows the results of male-to-male (two unrelated samples) hybridization. This experiment validated two measures: reproducibility and specificity. In each array, each BAC is spotted down in duplicate and each sample is hybridized twice, reversing the Cy3 and Cy5 labeling. This controls for dye-related labeling bias. Therefore, at each specific chromosome position (BAC), there are four data points. Each slide is then globally normalized such that the summed Cy3 signal equals the summed Cy5 signal. In order for a BAC to be identified as significantly differentially represented, the fluorescent intensities of the BAC duplicates are averaged and must show a change greater than two standard deviations (SD) over the normal control. This then has to be reproduced in the dye reversal experiment for the data point to be categorized as significantly differentially represented between the two samples. As expected, in the five replicate experiments that compared male-to-male hybridizations, no BAC clones reached these stringent criteria of being significantly differentially represented. This demonstrates the high degree of reproducibility of the arrays and gives strong evidence that false-positive changes will be very rare.

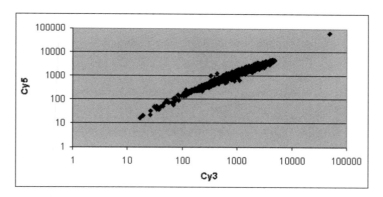

Figure 10-3. Scatter plot of male-to-male hybridizations. These data points represent the summed fluorescent intensities for the duplicate BAC clones. Note the strong linear correlation between the Cy3 and cy5 values. (*n*-5)

Figure 10-4 shows the male-to-female hybridization results and indicates the X dosage variation. The intensity of the X chromosome in the males never reached a value as low as 1.0 (ranges from 1.2-1.4). We postulate that this is due in part to the pseudoautosomal regions on the Y chromosome that carry X material[23]. But overall, the detection of females (XX) was readily observed when compared to males (XY). A consistent detection of a two-fold, single copy difference (one X chromosome [male] versus two X chromosomes [female]) shows the sensitivity of BAC microarrays. Therefore, the BAC arrays have the sensitivity to detect single copy deletion events.

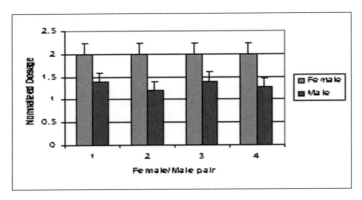

Figure 4. Four female/male pairs hybridized to BAC arrays for X chromosome dosage analysis. The sensitivity of this system is demonstrated by the consistent detection of the two-fold difference in X chromosome copy number. (*n*=5)

10.10 Conclusions

With the advent of microarray technology and its application to BAC arrays, researchers will now have the ability to analyze the entire genome at an unprecedented level of resolution. This will have a profound impact on studying how the genome can effect gene expression and phenotype and ultimately BAC arrays may become the workhorse for the cytogenetics and molecular diagnostic clinical laboratory.

The hardware for image aquistion of BAC arrays is the same as the scanners used for expression cDNA and printed oligo microarrays. The analysis of these images is greatly enhanced by the specialized software SpectralWare.

Acknowledgements

We would like to thank our collaborators at Texas Children's Hospital, Baylor College of Medicine, Albert Einstein College of Medicine, and University of California.

References

1. **Pandita A, Zielenska M, Thorner P, Bayani J, Godbout R, Greenberg M, Squire JA:** Application of comparative genomic hybridization, spectral karyotyping, and microarray analysis in the identification of subtype-specific patterns of genomic changes in rhabdomyosarcoma. *Neoplasia* 1999;1:262-275.

2. **Albertson DG, Ylstra B, Segraves R, Collins C, Dairkee SH, Kowbel D, Kuo WL, Gray JW, Pinkel D:** Quantitative mapping of amplicon structure by array CGH identifies CYP24 as a candidate oncogene. *Nat Genet* 2000;25:144-146.

3. **Heiskanen M, Kononen J, Barlund M, Torhorst J, Sauter G, Kallioniemi A, Kallioniemi O:** CGH, cDNA and tissue microarray analysis implicate FGFR2 amplification in a small subset of breast tumors. *Anal Cell Pathol* 2001;22:229-234.

4. **Pollack JR, Perou CM, Alizadeh AA, Eisen MB, Pergamenschikov A, Williams CF, Jeffrey SS, Botstein D, Brown PO:** Genome-wide analysis of DNA copy-number changes using cDNA microarrays. *Nat Genet* 1999;23:41-46.

5. **Takeo S, Arai H, Kusano N, Harada T, Furuya T, Kawauchi S, Oga A, Hirano T, Yoshida T, Okita K, Sasaki K:** Examination of oncogene amplification by genomic DNA microarray in hepatocellular carcinomas. comparison with comparative genomic hybridization analysis. *Cancer Genet Cytogenet* 2001;130:127-132.

6. **Browne CE, Dennis NR, Maher E, Long FL, Nicholson JC, Sillibourne J, Barber JC:** Inherited interstitial duplications of proximal 15q: genotype-phenotype correlations. *Am J Hum Genetics* 1997;61(6):1342-1352.

7. **Capone GT:** Down syndrome: advances in molecular biology and the neurosciences. *J Dev Behav Pediatr* 2001;22(1):40-59.

8. **Slamon DJ, Clark GM, Wong SG, Levin WJ, Ullrich A, McGuire WL:** Human breast cancer: correlation of relapse and survival with amplification of the HER-2/neu oncogene. *Science* 1987;235(4785):177-182.

9. **Collins C, Kuo WL, Segraves R, Fuscoe J, Pinkel D, and Gray JW**: Construction and characterization of plasmid libraries enriched in sequences from single human chromosomes. *Genomics* 1991;11(4):997-1006.

10. **Knight SJ, Horsley SW, Regan R, Lawrie NM, Maher EJ, Cardy DL, Flint J, and Kearney L:** Development and clinical application of an innovative fluorescence in situ hybridization technique which detects submicroscopic rearrangements involving telomeres. *Eur J Hum Genet* 1997;5(1):1-8.

11. **Speicher MR, Gwyn Ballard S, and Ward DC**: Karyotyping human chromosomes by combinatorial multi-fluor FISH. *Nat Genet* 1996;12(4):368-375.

12. **Schrock E, du Manoir S, Veldman T, Schoell B, Wienberg J, Ferguson-Smith MA, Ning Y, Ledbetter DH, Bar-Am I, Soenksen D, Garini Y, and Ried T:** Multicolor spectral karyotyping of human chromosomes. *Science* 1996;273(5274):494-497.

13. **Speicher MR and Ward DC:** The coloring of cytogenetics. *Nat Med* 1996;2(9):1046-1048.

14. **Kirchhoff M, Rose H, Lundsteen C:** High resolution comparative genomic hybridisation in clinical cytogenetics. *J Med Genet* 2001;38(11):740-4.

15. **Pinkel D, Segraves R, Sudar D, Clark S, Poole I, Kowbel D, Collins C, Kuo WL, Chen C, Zhai Y, Dairkee SH, Ljung BM, Gray JW, Albertson DG:** High resolution analysis of DNA copy number variation using comparative genomic hybridization to microarrays. *Nat Genet* 1998;20:207-211.

16. **Lander ES, Linton LM, Birren B, Nusbaum C, Zody MC, Baldwin J, Devon K, Dewar K, Doyle M, FitzHugh W, et al:** Initial sequencing and analysis of the human genome. *Nature* 2001;409(6822):860-921.

17. **Venter JC, Adams MD, Myers EW, Li PW, Mural RJ, Sutton GG, Smith HO, Yandell M, Evans CA, Holt RA, et al:** The sequence of the human genome. *Science* 2001;291(5507):1304-1351.

18. **Garson JA, van den Berghe JA, Kemshead JT:** Novel non-isotopic in situ hybridization technique detects small (1 Kb) unique sequences in routinely G-banded human chromosomes: fine mapping of N-myc and beta-NGF genes. *Nucleic Acids Res* 1987;15:4761-4770.

19. **Lichter P, Cremer T, Tang CJ, Watkins PC, Manuelidis L, Ward DC:** *Proc Natl Acad Sci USA* 1988;85:9664-9668.

20. **Kallioniemi A, Kallioniemi OP, Sudar D, Rutovitz D, Gray JW, Waldman F, Pinkel D:** Comparative genomic hybridization for molecular cytogenetic analysis of solid tumors. *Science* 1992;258:818-821.

21. **Cheung VG, Nowak N, Jang W, Kirsch IR, Zhao S, Chen XN, Furey TS, Kim UJ, Kuo WL, Olivier M, et al:** Integration of cytogenetic landmarks into the draft sequence of the human genome. *Nature* 2001;409(6822):953-958.

22. **McPherson JD, Marra M, Hillier L, Waterston RH, Chinwalla A, Wallis J, Sekhon M, Wylie K, Mardis ER, Wilson RK, et al:** A physical map of the human genome. *Nature* 2001;409(6822):934-941).

23. **Geschwind DH, Gregg J, Boone K, Karrim J, Pawlikowska-Haddal A, Rao E, Ellison J, Ciccodicola A, D'Urso M, Woods R, Rappold GA, Swerdloff R, and Nelson SF:** Klinefelter's syndrome as a model of anomalous cerebral laterality: testing gene dosage in the X chromosome pseudoautosomal region using a DNA microarray. *Dev Genet* 1998;23(3):215-222.

INDEX

shape regularity 120-121
flagging 122
perimeter 120
background 137
Stationary random field 24
Sub-grid 10, 100
t-test 116

Transfer function 25

Wavelet transforms 22
Wiener filtering 24

Xenon lamp 56

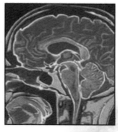
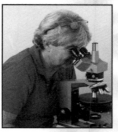
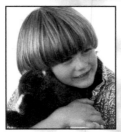
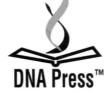

ORDER FORM

To order books in bulk at discount, please complete this form and fax the entire page back to DNA Press at **501-694-5495**. E-mail **dnapress@yahoo.com** if you have any questions. Attn: Xela Schenk, Operations Manager. *Price of one book: $29.95*

TITLE (DESCRIPTION)	QUANTITY	PRICE PER BOOK	SUBTOTAL (quantity x price)
MICROARRAY IMAGE ANALYSIS: NUTS & BOLTS October 2002; ISBN 0-9664027-5-8 5-10 books		$22.00	$
MICROARRAY IMAGE ANALYSIS: NUTS & BOLTS October 2002; ISBN 0-9664027-5-8 10-30 books		$18.00	$
MICROARRAY IMAGE ANALYSIS: NUTS & BOLTS October 2002; ISBN 0-9664027-5-8 more than 30 books		$15.00	$
SHIPPING & HANDLING COSTS **Within North America:** $10 for 5-10 books - book rate $15 for 10-30 books - 2nd day	Shipping & Handling		$
	Subtotal		$
Outside North America: $15 for 5-30 books - standard	5% PA. Sales Tax		$
$20 for 5-30 books - express	**TOTAL**		$

Method of payment:

☐ Check   *(Make payable to DNAPress, P.O. Box 572, Eagleville, PA 19408)*

☐ Please bill us   ☐ Visa   ☐ Mastercard   ☐ AmericanExpress

Card # _____   Exp. Date: _____/_____

Cardholder Signature: _____

Name: _____

Job Title: _____

Signature: _____

Organization: _____

Shipping Address: _____

City/State/Zip: _____

Phone: _____   Ext: _____

Fax: _____   E-mail *(Required)*: _____

Notes: